Safeguarding and Mental Health Support in Contemporary Childhood

Approaches regarding safeguarding and mental health in childhood have been in constant flux. Framed within a critical realist ontology, this book provides insight into causal factors (individual, material, institutional) and social structures that impact on the continued legacy of the 'deserving/undeserving' paradigm.

Drawing on historical data from children taken into care by the Waifs and Strays Society (1881–1918) and contemporary data from interviews with young care leavers and safeguarding practitioners/professionals, this book shows how at present and in the past, certain children and families miss(ed) out on support and interventions due to complex needs, financial cuts and ever-changing thresholds. It is the group of children referred to as 'victims', a term used for the most disadvantaged children who have spent time in care, have complex mental health needs and have had the most damaging pre-care family experiences, who are the focus of this book. This book shows that in an attempt to provide services where there are ever-increasing thresholds for access and cuts to resources, a resurgence of the 'deserving/undeserving' paradigm reflects a contemporary justification regarding who is 'entitled' to help and who is not.

This book will be of interest to all scholars and students of social work, social policy, childhood studies, sociology and education policy.

Wendy Sims-Schouten is Associate Professor (Reader) in Childhood Studies, School of Education and Sociology, University of Portsmouth, UK.

Safeguarding and Mental Health Support in Contemporary Childhood

How the Deserving/Undeserving Paradigm from the Past Overshadows the Present

Wendy Sims-Schouten

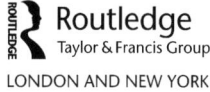
Routledge
Taylor & Francis Group

LONDON AND NEW YORK

First published 2021
by Routledge
2 Park Square, Milton Park, Abingdon, Oxon OX14 4RN

and by Routledge
52 Vanderbilt Avenue, New York, NY 10017

Routledge is an imprint of the Taylor & Francis Group, an informa business

British Library Cataloguing in Publication Data
A catalogue record for this book is available from the British Library

Library of Congress Cataloging-in-Publication Data
Names: Sims-Schouten, Wendy, author.
Title: Safeguarding and mental health support in contemporary childhood : how the deserving/undeserving paradigm from the past overshadows the present / Wendy Sims-Schouten.
Description: Milton Park, Abingdon, Oxon ; New York, NY : Routledge, 2021. | Includes bibliographical references and index.
Identifiers: LCCN 2020031316 (print) | LCCN 2020031317 (ebook) | ISBN 9780367000912 (hardback) | ISBN 9780429444555 (ebook)
Subjects: LCSH: Child health services. | Child abuse–Prevention. | Child mental health. | Children–Social aspects. | Families–Economic aspects.
Classification: LCC RJ101 .S524 2021 (print) | LCC RJ101 (ebook) | DDC 362.19892–dc23
LC record available at https://lccn.loc.gov/2020031316
LC ebook record available at https://lccn.loc.gov/2020031317

ISBN: 978-0-367-00091-2 (hbk)
ISBN: 978-0-429-44455-5 (ebk)

Typeset in Times New Roman
by Taylor & Francis Books

To Julian and Celeste for their love and encouragement!

Contents

Tables

Introduction
Setting the scene

Mary was six years old when, in 1892, she was taken on by the Waifs and Strays Society, one of Britain's largest child care agencies from the late 19th century to the present day, and sent to a children's home in Hampshire in the UK. Her mother had died of cancer when Mary was four, and her dad lived in a workhouse and was sentenced to three months' imprisonment for neglect. Between 1892 and 1907 Mary spent time in various institutions – a children's home, a mental hospital, as well as a country asylum and the workhouse. Correspondence linked to her case comes from a range of sources, including a medical officer and various people linked to the institutions where Mary resided, as well as correspondence from Mary herself. For example, in 1898 the children's home refers to Mary as 'having no control over herself and at times very violent', while correspondence from a county asylum in 1900 refers to her 'weak intellect' and describes her as 'silly and childish in behaviour and very idle'. There is reference to her being insane, and that 'this case will inevitably have to be dealt with by the Poor Law authorities'. Yet, there is also a caring tone to some of the correspondence from carers who 'have concern for her and are anxious to stay in touch' and the 'After Care Association', whose correspondence refers to Mary as being 'a nice girl and should do well, if only her mental condition remains satisfactory'. Correspondence from Mary herself shows a girl who is very articulate but also aware of the issues around her; she indicates 'I know I have a lot to be thankful for' and (referring to her attempted suicide) 'I know I did a very mad act.'

Fast forward 124 years, and Jake has been in care since he was three years old. He is currently 21 years old and has spent time in various children's homes, as well as in foster care. He is no longer in touch with his foster family since he has become an adult and moved away into supported accommodation. He suffers from panic attacks, and describes his mental health as 'extremely complicated' and 'something that has gone on for an extremely long time'. He is lonely and refers to not having any friends, and that he 'hates change' and 'new people'. Yet, he also refers to himself as difficult – 'I can be quite difficult you know' – and grateful for the after-care support he is receiving as 'it helps me to have at least a person to talk to'. Interviews with safeguarding practitioners flag up something else, namely that 'Jake had a rough time in care and just needs someone to support him'; it also shows that they are stretched and at times unable or even unwilling to support children with complex needs, and one care worker highlights 'we can't support young people like Jake'.

This book focuses on young people like Mary and Jake, the group of children referred to by Mike Stein (2006) as 'victims' – a term used for the most disadvantaged children who have spent time in care, have complex needs and have had the most damaging pre-care family experiences. Their time in care is characterised by further difficulties, instability and disruption. After leaving care they are likely to be unemployed and become homeless, to be lonely and isolated and have mental health problems. The starting point for this research is the notion that many of the issues that concern contemporary studies regarding child safeguarding and child protection have a historical trajectory that informs the present (see also Hacking, 1991; Stainton Rogers & Stainton Rogers, 1992). Definitions and conceptions in relation to mental health, abuse and neglect in childhood have been in constant flux and need to be seen in light of the complexities and confusions of history (Cradock, 2014; Hacking, 1991). As such, what we mean by child abuse and neglect and related safeguarding measures is not a reflection of the current state of knowledge, but rather a legacy inherited from the 19th-century child rescue movement.

What both Mary and Jake have in common is their personal history of being in the care system, as well as their material context, placing them on the margins of society with no privileges at all. They both indicate that they are grateful and appreciative of the (albeit limited) help and support received, whilst also referring to themselves as 'doing a mad act' or 'being difficult'. Their social position could, therefore, be understood as providing the 'scaffolding' for their positive construction of the input of the care worker/children's home as it reflects their (real and perceived) lack of entitlement. Not only that, but the focus on their 'bad behaviour' hints at the fact that in the greater scheme of things they are not all that 'deserving' of the help and support they so desperately need. Yet, this negates the fact that, due to their pre-care experiences and related trauma, looked after children can have challenging emotional and behavioural difficulties, as a result of which a significant number of placements break down and children experience numerous placements (Fisher et al., 2000; Hardwick, 2005). However, whilst some may class their behaviour as 'disordered' and 'delinquent', it could also be argued that what they show is an attempt to function, survive and be resilient through the only means available to them (Ungar, 2002, 2004, 2005).

Mary grew up in a time that was marked by a purge on spending on the poor, stimulated by the New Poor Law of 1834 through which a system of 'deservedness' was introduced (King, 2018; MacKinnon, 1987). Here the poor 'deserving of help' were considered as the ones who had become poor through no fault of their own, such as through bereavement or being frail and elderly, whilst the poor labelled as 'undeserving of help' were the 'lazy' ones, the 'criminal' and 'able-bodied' (Shore, 2003). Yet, this decision was highly subjective, and 'bad behaviour' and 'mental inferiority' were also used to class certain groups of people as undeserving, and it could be argued that Mary falls within this group. Jake, from the present time, also appears to be judged by his behaviour and classed as 'undeserving' of help.

The key questions here (and the focus of this book) are: what mechanisms and causal factors are at play, and what is the legacy of the 'deserving/undeserving' paradigm in mental health support and safeguarding in childhood? The research is driven by a critical realist informed, stratified model of reality. Applying a critical realist approach means taking account of the fact that practices and perceptions, in this case with a focus on child safeguarding and mental health support, are both socially constructed and influenced by external factors and forces that can be real and independent of any one person or social group (see also Sims-Schouten et al., 2019).

This book consists of five chapters and a conclusion. The first chapter – entitled 'Safeguarding, mental health and the legacy of the "deserving/undeserving" paradigm: worthy or unworthy victims?' – provides an overview of the development of child safeguarding and mental health support practices in the UK. The chapter specifically focuses on developments and practices since the implementation of the New Poor Law of 1834 through to contemporary times. As well as shedding light on the workings of the 'deserving/undeserving' paradigm, Chapter 1 will also provide insights into dominant practices and perceptions in relation to child safeguarding, mental health, wellbeing and mental illness in childhood, and key concepts such as 'lunatic', 'imbecile' and 'wretched families'. It will also explore how historic practices, such as in relation to child guidance clinics, have fed into the welfare state and the creation and establishment of the National

Health Service (NHS) in 1948. The chapter ends with a reflection on the legacy of the deserving/undeserving paradigm through time.

Chapter 2, 'Mental health and safeguarding through a critical realist lens', provides a critical route through the varied, sometimes confusing and contradictory, maze of practices and perceptions of psychiatrists, psychologists and social workers, all of which have evolved from different routes and ontologies. The chapter proposes critical realism as an approach that brings together the range of epistemologies and ontologies of the varying disciplines, combining a general philosophy of science with a philosophy of social science to describe an interface between the natural and social worlds. Critical realism invites us to adopt a form of reasoning called 'retroduction', which involves moving from the level of observation and lived experiences to making (non-linear) inferences about underlying structures and mechanisms that may account for the phenomena involved. In Chapter 2 I will explain how, drawing on critical realist ontology and retroduction, it is possible to provide insight into a stratified model of reality, allowing us to conceptualise the 'real' (exploring causal mechanisms of events), the 'empirical' (experienced events) and the 'actual' (events and processes that occur). This is especially relevant in relation to making sense of the complexities surrounding safeguarding and mental health in childhood. Chapter 2 not only provides insights into the benefits of applying critical realism to this context, but also how this works in practice, analysing material from historic and contemporary datasets.

The historic dataset comprises case files of children taken into care by the Waifs and Strays Society from its inception in 1881 through to 1918, and will be discussed in Chapter 3. Over 22,000 children from across England and Wales were cared for by the Society between 1881 and the end of the First World War. The children's case files consist of correspondence highlighting the perception of custodians, educators, medical officers, clergymen, practitioners linked to asylums and industrial schools, parents and children (during and after care). Drawing on critical realism and thematic content analysis of 108 children's case files, the chapter will provide insights into perceptions and conditions in relation to the safeguarding and mental health of the most vulnerable children of the time.

Chapter 4, entitled 'The case of care leavers, mental health and safeguarding in contemporary Britain', puts the experiences of said young care leavers into perspective, drawing on the voice of the most vulnerable care leavers, referred to by Stein (2006) as 'victims'. As with Chapter 3, Chapter 4 draws on critical realist ontology, specifically the notion of retroduction and stratified non-linear dynamics of embodied experiences, material/institutional forces and social relationships that co-constitute subjectivity, to make sense experiences. A total of 46 participants were interviewed: 24 were care leavers and 22 were safeguarding practitioners; and, as with Chapter 3, data was analysed using thematic content analysis.

Chapter 5 – 'Good practice and bad practice: lessons learnt' – summarises the key findings in relation to the historic and contemporary datasets presented in Chapters 3 and 4, and provides examples of good and bad practices with vulnerable children and young people, identifying ways forward. The chapter starts with a reflection on the legacy of the deserving/undeserving paradigm in practice with vulnerable children, as well concepts such as that some children are 'beyond help'. Here I also reflect on challenges in multi-agency team work, and perceptions in relation to 'problem children' and whose 'job' it is to support those children. In addition to this, I will reflect on 'childhood' and what this means to different children from different eras, cultural contexts and ethnicities, leading into a discussion regarding the legacy of trauma: the latter is often overlooked, i.e. the notion that neglect and abuse have transgenerational as well as intergenerational impacts, just like the deserving/undeserving paradigm.

This book was made possible with a grant from the Wellcome Trust, for which I am very grateful. I am also grateful for the support of many colleagues, friends and family when it came to reading drafts and providing me with tea and coffee whilst I was writing the book. I would specifically like to thank my colleagues and friends Fran Salvi, Helen Haste and Helen Cowie for reading drafts of the chapters, as well as Steven Taylor for providing useful and positive feedback regarding my proposal, and Annie Skinner for being my buddy when I did my archival research at the Children's Society's archives in London. I would also like to thank the many people, agencies and charities who have supported me in collecting my data, too many to mention! Finally, I would like to thank my husband and daughter, for always being a listening ear for my sometimes wacky ideas and thoughts. Most of all I would like to thank the young people and practitioners who were part of my research; all of them have left their mark and my heart goes out to them.

References

Cradock, G. (2014). Who owns child abuse? *Social Sciences*, 3, 854–870.

Fisher, T., Gibbs, I., Sinclair, I. and Wilson, K. (2000). Sharing the care: the qualities sought of social workers by foster carers. *Child & Family Social Work*, 5(3), 225–233.

Hacking, I. (1991), The making and molding of child abuse. *Critical Inquiry*, 17(2), 253–288.

Hardwick, L. (2005), Fostering children with sexualised behaviour. *Adoption & Fostering*, 29(2), 33–43.

King, S.A. (2018). *Sickness, Medical Welfare and the English Poor 1750–1834*. Manchester: Manchester University Press.

MacKinnon, M. (1987). English Poor Law policy and the crusade against outdoor relief. *Journal of Economic History*, 47(3), 603–625.

Shore, H. (2003). Crime, criminal networks and the survival strategies of the poor in early eighteenth-century London. In: King, S. and Tomkins, A. (Eds.), *The Poor in England 1700–1850* (137–165). Manchester and New York: Manchester University Press.

Sims-Schouten, W., Skinner, A. and Rivett, K. (2019). Child safeguarding in light of the deserving/undeserving paradigm: a historical and contemporary analysis, *Child Abuse & Neglect*, 94, doi:10.1016/j.chiabu.2019.104025.

Stainton Rogers, W. and Stainton Rogers, R. (1992). *Stories of Childhood: Shifting Agendas of Child Concern*. New York: Harvester Wheatsheaf.

Stein, M. (2006). Research review: young people leaving care. *Child and Family Social Work*, 11, 273–279.

Ungar, M. (2002). *Playing at Being Bad: The Hidden Resilience of Troubled Teens*. East Lawrencetown, NS: Pottersfield Press.

Ungar, M. (2004). *Nurturing Hidden Resilience in Troubled Youth*. Toronto: University of Toronto Press.

Ungar, M. (2005). *A Handbook for Working with Children and Youth: Pathways to Resilience across Cultures and Contexts*. Thousand Oaks, CA: Sage.

1 Safeguarding, mental health and the legacy of the 'deserving/undeserving' paradigm

Worthy or unworthy victims?

In this chapter I will outline and discuss the development of child safeguarding and mental health support practices in the UK, including perceptions around 'deserving/undeserving' children and those who 'can be helped' or are 'beyond help'. Contemporary approaches towards safeguarding and mental health support in childhood should be seen in light of the complex interaction between beliefs, ideologies and practices inherited from the English Poor Law legislation (which can be traced back to 1536); the child rescue movement and early children's homes – with the establishment in 1739 of the Foundling Hospital, the first English charity devoted exclusively to children; and child psychology/psychiatry (Higginbotham, 2017; King, 2018; Taylor, 2016).

The main focus of the chapter is on developments from the 1800s onwards; but I will also touch on earlier developments, such as the Poor Law of 1601, which introduced a basic social security system. Moreover, this chapter will discuss the development of the child rescue movement in the late 1800s, child guidance clinics in the 1900s and the establishment in 1948 of the NHS and the welfare state. As well as focusing on the development of practice, I will also highlight how practices, with a specific focus on the last 150 years, have been influenced by the legacy of the 'deserving/undeserving' paradigm. The main purpose of this chapter is to provide an overview of social care practices and mental health support introduced from late Victorian times to the present day, highlighting that, despite the numerous acts, policies and developments in practice, there is still a long way to go when it comes to supporting the most vulnerable children in society.

1.1 The deserving/undeserving paradigm and the child rescue movement

This section will discuss what role the deserving/undeserving paradigm played in decisions around child protection and the child rescue movement of the late 1800s, which is foundational to social work as we know it today. The New Poor Law (covering England and Wales), which 'legalised' the notion of 'deservedness', represented a system of poor relief that was in existence until the establishment of the modern welfare state in 1948 (King, 2003; MacKinnon, 1987). The New Poor Law, introduced in 1834, was implemented to reduce spending on the poor by centralising the notion of 'deservedness'. It did so by embracing a notion of eligibility: the idea that some people are deserving of welfare support due to an inability to work through no fault of their own. These included the old, the infirm, widows, children and those who found themselves temporarily out of work due to the cyclical nature of the rural economy, with its peaks and troughs of employment needs (Atherton, 2011; King, 2019; Royden, 2017). At the same time, those who were capable of working but chose not to do so were regarded as undeserving and were ineligible for support; although it should be noted here that in the past, just as it is presently, judgements around work 'capability' and 'choice' were largely subjective (Sales, 2002; Skinner & Thomas, 2018). Support was given as outdoor relief, where claimants were allowed to continue to live in their own homes, and indoor relief through admission to the workhouse. The latter could be harsh, and was perceived as a form of punishment for the undeserving poor due to the imposed compulsory labour and residence in the workhouse (Carter et al., 2019).

The history of the Poor Law in England and Wales (as this developed slightly differently in Scotland) is usually separated into two statutes: the Old Poor Law, which was passed during the reign of Elizabeth I; and the New Poor Law, passed in 1834 – the latter significantly modified the existing system of poor relief (King, 2018). The notion of 'deservedness' was at the heart of welfare practices and support stimulated by the Old Poor Law from its codification in 1597 and 1601, and developed into a more punitive form following the New Poor Law (Croll, 2017; MacKinnon, 1987).

The 1601 codification act implemented the Old Poor Law and formed the legal basis for efforts to protect needy adults and children through *parens patriae* (parent of the nation), the public policy power to intervene against a negligent parent. This was administered haphazardly and arbitrarily at local parish level, subject to the generosity of relief, leaving it up to local administrators to decide who was deserving and who was not, and led to stark variations in local practice (King, 2003; Roberts, 1963; Schene 1998).

In contrast, the New Poor Law of 1834 marked a highly centralised system that encouraged the large-scale development of workhouses by

Poor Law Unions. As such, the New Poor Law could be perceived as more punitive than the Old Poor Law as the former introduced a principle of 'less eligibility', resulting in a much less flexible method of providing poor relief than before (Atherton, 2011; Price, 2012). Under the leadership of George Goschen, president of the Poor Law Board, a 'crusade' was introduced that slashed Poor Law spending in 1869 (Hurren, 2015), and some argue that this marked the implementation of the 1834 Poor Law Act (Croll, 2017; Skinner & Thomas, 2018). The Charity Organisation Society (COS) was established in 1869 and worked with the Poor Law authorities to develop a system of personal social work to increase effectiveness among charities and to organise charitable giving (Hurren, 2015; Thane, 2012). Goschen suggested that the Poor Law should deal with the undeserving and the guardians of the newly founded COS the deserving (Strand, 2016). This shift in cost-cutting can be seen as foundational to the social work that grew from it and, perhaps, even as an early example of the state outsourcing care of children to private interests.

The latter half of the 19th century saw the rise of the child rescue movement and philanthropic voluntary agencies providing institutional care and support for the poor, destitute and orphaned young. At this time, child safeguarding in the UK was organised through a combination of state support and philanthropic voluntary agencies; one example of a voluntary organisation was the Waifs and Strays Society (now known as the Children's Society), established in 1881 by Edward Rudolf (Higginbotham, 2017; Taylor, 2015, 2016). The Charity Organisation Society guardians were active across the UK, and were encouraged to join other voluntary organisations (such as institutions providing residential child care services) that helped the poor and influenced them to change their behaviour (Hendrick, 1994; Skinner & Thomas, 2018). The COS was involved in the Waifs and Strays Society from early on, as it was keen to influence organisations in their policies (Sims-Schouten et al., 2019; Skinner & Thomas, 2018). Yet, whilst child philanthropy developed, providing child care services as an alternative to the workhouse, Government welfare policy was focused on separating the deserving from the undeserving, encouraging self-help and changing behaviour (Sohasky, 2015; Skinner & Thomas, 2018; Taylor, 2015).

Child philanthropy and the child rescue movement need to be seen in light of this complex interaction and relationship between and the history of concepts and ideologies around poverty, the criminal mind and the 'mad'. Although the notion of deservedness was used to distinguish the lazy, idle poor from the poor who had met with misfortune (e.g. the death of a husband, disability, etc.), the interpretation was essentially subjective. It should also be noted that across the UK there were differences in the way in which the Poor Law Acts were applied. For example, unlike in England, the Scottish poor had the right to appeal decisions made under the New Poor Law, which came into existence in Scotland in 1845 (Keane, 1987). This is also reflected in admissions to children's homes/institutions. For example, admissions to the Waifs and Strays' homes (from 1881) in England were based on appeals by church representatives, while admissions to the Royal Scottish Institute for 'mentally impaired' children (from 1862) were based on judgements by the governors regarding the deservedness of the child (Hurren, 2015; Strand, 2016; Ward, 1990).

While on the surface 'the poor man/woman/child' (honest and industrious), 'the criminal' (disorderly and immoral) and 'the insane' (mentally ill) are not easy bedfellows, I argue that it is in the way in which their lives overlapped and the inability/unwillingness of the middle classes to distinguish between the three that the ongoing influence of the deserving/undeserving paradigm can be seen in historic and contemporary approaches and practices. These were adults (and their children) who walked the same paths between home, lodgings, unemployment, poor relief, charity and workhouse, instigating judgements around deservedness (King, 2018, 2019; Shore, 2003). This can be seen, for example, in the writings of Victorian journalist Henry Mayhew (1812–1887), who produced a series of newspaper articles for the *Morning Chronicle* (a newspaper published between 1769 and 1862) describing the state of the London poor. The articles, published in 1851, were later compiled into a book entitled *London Labour and the London Poor*, published in numerous editions (Mayhew, 1968, 2008, 2010; see also Taithe, 1996). In volume one (1968) Mayhew wrote: 'I shall consider the whole of the metropolitan poor under three separate phases, according as they will work, they can't work, and they won't work.' Moreover, with his publications Mayhew also drew attention to how marginal and precarious many people's lives were in what, at that time (the mid to late 1800s), was the richest city in the world (Mayhew, 1968; Münch, 2018, Taithe, 1996).

Yet, whilst journalists like Henry Mayhew and others, such as James Greenwood (1832–1923), drew attention to the way the poor people of London lived and worked, there is evidence that fears from the middle and upper classes that their comfortable moral and economic situation would be threatened were becoming more intense (Stedman Jones, 1971). This coincided with a slash on public spending by the Government from 1869, restricting the provision of material support and outdoor relief (Skinner & Thomas, 2018; Thane, 2012). This purge on spending on the poor in the late 1800s was followed by and co-occurred with what is generally seen as the start of the child rescue movement: a time when numerous philanthropists – such as Thomas Barnardo, Edward Rudolf and John Throgmorton Middlemore, to name a few – opened homes for poor and destitute children. All were motivated by the desire to protect poor and abandoned children, and saving them from an institutional upbringing in the workhouse by providing them with a 'family environment' through placements in homes and foster care (Higginbotham, 2017). Yet, the notion of 'deservedness' had left its mark, and the deserving/undeserving paradigm played a significant role in decisions around which children should and shouldn't be supported; this will be discussed in more detail in the next section.

1.2 'Earnest solicitation', 'terrible suffering' or a 'pest to society'?

Childhood and childhood experience were at the heart of much philanthropic work in the late Victorian era, and voluntary organisations such as the Waifs and Strays Society encouraged donors to empathise with poor children (Moruzi, 2017). One way in which this was done was through advertisements in periodicals. *Aunt Judy's Magazine*, a middle-class monthly founded in 1866 by Margaret Gatty and aimed at a readership of both boys and girls, is an example of this (Gatty, 1871; Rauch, 1997). In 1871 *Aunt Judy's Magazine* appealed to its readers to raise money for a cot for the Great Ormond Street Hospital for Sick Children (GOSH) in London, taking advantage of the charitable impulses of the time. As an example, correspondence in the Christmas volume of that year includes the following:

> It was intended that the 'Cot' should be removed into the girls' ward for the New Year, but the transfer has been postponed in order to accede to the earnest solicitation of a poor little boy, whose illness causes terrible suffering, and who begged so hard to be Aunt Judy's patient, that it was felt impossible to refuse his request (p. 127).

The portrayal of the 'earnest solicitation' of the 'poor little boy' exposed to 'terrible suffering' and 'begging so hard to be Aunt Judy's patient' is interesting in this light, highlighting that 'deservedness', 'worthiness' and 'sincerity' are inherent in support decisions. This ambiguous and tricky relationship and distinction between the institutions of poor relief and the wider world can also be seen in other parts of Europe, such as France (Dobbin, 1994; Gelfand, 1984). Moreover, for some, faced with a highly subjective system of poor relief, theft was one of the more lucrative means of sustaining oneself (Carter et al., 2019; King, 2003). While this would class them as 'delinquent' and 'disordered', it could also be argued that this behaviour signifies a hidden pathway to resilience, i.e. the capacity to overcome adversity through the only means available to them (Ungar, 2002, 2004, 2005).

A striking similarity can be seen not only in the way in which public spending on the poor and vulnerable is slashed in the second half of the 19th century and the present time, but also between calls from the press to reduce state help and promote voluntarism both in Victorian times and today's Western society. For example, whilst an article in *The Times* on 1 January 1876 refers to 'indiscriminate charity making bad parents and bad parents create a greater demand for indiscriminate charity', on 4 September 2013 an article in the *Mail* stressed that 'even claimants admit they are getting too much in benefits: 59 per cent of those given handouts think they discourage work' (Groves, 2013). Thus, in both the Victorian era and contemporary times people in need of benefits and support were and are stigmatised, placing them on the margins of society, with little regard for the cause or consequence and/ or issues around wellbeing and trauma (Cromby & Harper, 2009; Taylor, 2016, Cox, 2013). Moreover, the 'harsh Victorian times' are often used as a reference when criticising current practices in relation to welfare and charity work. For example, on 28 February 2017 *The Guardian* newspaper published an anonymous article with the heading 'As a charity boss, I despair of Victorian attitudes ruining our good work', whilst an article from the same newspaper of 20 July 2017 highlighted that 'Critics condemn the "Victorian approach" to treatment of mental health patients' (Campbell, 2017).

It should however be noted that the image of the uncaring and emotionally distant Victorians does not necessarily reflect the ideology and practice of the time; and, as with current practices and ideologies, it is crucial to see this in light of different institutional, religious and philanthropic approaches (Moss et al., 2017). For example, alongside calls to abandon 'indiscriminate charity', the Victorian press also alludes to a need for more support and awareness regarding child protection and care. An article in *The Guardian* in December 1892 calls out for a need for 'more philanthropy and public help'. Similarly, in contemporary news items there are calls for support and suggestions that 'We are failing our children' (DeGarmo, 2015), as well as evidence to the contrary. An example of this is the ambiguous portrayal of 'callous and unemotional' children in the media (e.g. in the *New York*

Times, Psychology Today and *Daily Mail Australia*), as if this is a given and some children are just 'born bad' (see Khan, 2012; Bergland, 2017; Huffadine, 2015).

By the mid to late 1800s there were a multitude of institutions in Britain that were used as substitutes for children's 'natural' homes, from orphanages (although it should be noted that these institutions also largely catered for children who weren't orphans) to a wide range of other establishments run by charities, religious groups, workhouse authorities, local councils and single individuals serving particular purposes (e.g. moral protection, penal confinement, etc.) (Higginbotham, 2017; King 2003; Skinner & Thomas, 2018). Alongside the development of industrial schools in the mid to late 1800s (born out of the reformatories and ragged schools) for the moral improvement of destitute, homeless and thieving youth was the introduction of lunatic asylums to Britain. It should however be noted that while the modern era of institutionalised provision for the care of the mentally ill began in the early 19th century, prompted by the 1808 County Asylums Act, London's Bethlem (or Bedlam) Royal Hospital – Europe's oldest extant psychiatric hospital – had operated continuously for over 600 years (Andrews et al., 1997; Higginbotham, 2017).

Asylums originated in France in the 17th century, and were institutions that symbolised progress and therapeutic optimism, as well as being instruments of social control where the poor and incurable could be swept out of sight (Arnold, 2008). Few references can be found with a focus on psychiatry, psychopathology and mental health in childhood prior to the 19th century. That is not to say that children weren't institutionalised; on the contrary, there is evidence that children were admitted to Bethlem Hospital and county asylums (Gingell, 2001; Wilkins, 1987). Yet, children were treated much the same here as adult patients, and as such there is no evidence that asylums contributed significantly to the development of the disciplines of social work, child psychology and child psychiatry. The first attempt to develop a coordinated strategy with a focus on mental health and safeguarding in childhood did not develop until the 20th century (Cradock, 2014; Hacking, 1991); this will be discussed in more detail below.

1.3 'Lunatic', 'imbecile' and 'wretched families'

Practices and perceptions regarding mental health/mental illness and safeguarding in childhood need to be viewed in light of dominant conceptualisations embraced by different generations of professionals/ practitioners, theorists and social classes, stimulated by social, economic, religious and political challenges of their respective eras (Cradock, 2014; Hendrick, 1997). Down through the decades, theorists, professionals and politicians have set the stage for various viewpoints regarding practices concerning child protection, mental health support and safeguarding in childhood. As mentioned earlier, there is evidence that children spent time in asylums long before there was any interest in or acknowledgement of childhood as a separate stage of development, and children were treated the same as the adult patients. Asylums as such did not contribute significantly to the development of the discipline of child psychiatry, psychology and social work (Gingell, 2001). Similarly, it is not possible to equate historic diagnoses of 'mental deficiency' or 'imbecility' (among others) with recognisable contemporary diagnoses. The dominant perception of the time was that children were born without reason, and as such could not 'lose their mind' or 'go mad'. For example, Henry Maudsley – a pioneering British psychiatrist of the late 1800s and founder of the eponymous psychiatric hospital in London in 1907 – asserted that a child cannot go 'mad', due to not having a mind to go wrong (Maudsley, 1879). Common diagnoses for those under the age of ten included 'idiocy' and 'imbecility', but did not necessarily indicate cognitive deficiencies. Instead, 'idiocy' was seen as an example of reversion to a lower level on the evolutionary scale. The general view was that children's minds and their ability to reason would develop gradually as they grew into adults; as such, children could not then, by definition, be insane (Melling et al., 1997; Taylor, 2016).

Although there is evidence that some children in every era have shown emotional and behavioural problems (e.g. the first writings about abnormal behaviour in childhood can be seen in early Greece), up until the 20th century behavioural disorders were largely considered moral issues and problems: the result of 'badness' rather than 'madness', and deserving of punishment (Mash & Wolfe, 2019). Similarly, until recently failure to learn did not necessarily indicate cognitive deficiencies, and instead could result in a marginalised existence, for example as a village idiot; 'idiocy' and 'imbecility' were common diagnoses for those under the age of ten (Sohasky, 2015).

Regardless of the full meaning of 'imbecility' and the possible overlap between this and 'insanity' and 'madness' – e.g. Maudsley's book dedicated a chapter to 'the insanity of early life', while Griesinger (1867) noted that mania and melancholia did occur in children – it is evident that two overarching causal factors were ascribed to 'abnormality' in children in the 19th century. First, there were psychological causes, such as fright and grief; and, second, there were physical causes, including epilepsy and infectious fevers like typhoid and measles (Parry-Jones, 1972). Evidence of this can be found in historic case files and archives from the second half of that century, such as those of the Royal Scottish National Institution (a facility for 'mentally impaired' children, established in 1862). Applications from 1864 to 1892 highlight that anything from 'a sudden fright from a bull calf' through to scarlet fever, epilepsy and 'marital age of the parents' were among the causal factors attributed to 'imbecility'. Moreover, 'imbecility' itself is discussed here in terms of 'violent outbursts' and 'dullness', as well as a 'mental condition' and 'the violence of God'. Thus, although psychological and physical causes of abnormality in children are starting to be recognised from the late 1800s, there is (still) little acknowledgement of the fact that behavioural and emotional issues can be a function of abuse and related mental health problems (Cradock, 2014; Hacking, 1991).

At the same time, from the end of the 19th century, it became more widely acknowledged that juvenile insanity and 'madness' in children was different from 'mental retardation' and epilepsy (Sampson, 1976; Rey et al., 2015; Stewart, 2011). The notion of 'development' became a key concept surrounding the study of children and childhood (Prout & James, 1997), with some developmental stages being construed as more problematic than others. For example, puberty became recognised as a causal factor in insanity: American psychiatrist Benjamin Rush referred to 'masturbation insanity' in children, and in 1889 French physician Maxime Durand-Fardel highlighted the existence of suicide in children (Rey et al., 2015). Medical doctor George Shuttleworth (1903) refers to 'morbid sexual erethism' as one of the 'slighter forms of mental defect in children', which may nevertheless lead to grave moral delinquencies and results from neuroticism and restless behaviour in early childhood, as well as neurotic parents and heredity. In the early 1900s there was a growing understanding of the multiple factors involved in the development of childhood psychiatric disorders, although the emphasis was predominantly on heredity. G. Stanley Hall, an American psychologist with a specific interest in child development and eugenics, made studying children a priority in science (Partridge 1912; Stewart, 2009). Hall's book on adolescence, published in 1904, was widely read across the Western world, including England, and drew attention to the role of heredity and environment in moral development and psychopathology in childhood. According to Hall (1904, 335, 338):

> Degenerate children are neurotic, irritable, vain, lacking in vigor, very fluctuating in mood, prone to aberrant tendencies under stress, often sexually perverted, with extreme shyness.

And

> Poverty and crime are closely correlated with starvation of body and mind, so that both are prone to arrest and both heredity and environment cooperate in producing modifications of physical structures and psychic powers.

This focus on psychopathology and heredity can also be seen in the language of the child guidance movement (which first emerged in the USA in the aftermath of the First World War, spreading to Britain and other parts of Europe shortly thereafter), which was suffused with medical terminology (Stewart, 2009, 2011). Led by a team consisting of three professions – psychiatry, psychology and psychiatric social work (although in reality this was very hierarchical, with the psychiatrist very much in charge) – child guidance clinics sought to be a form of preventive medicine promoting children's mental wellbeing and preventing mental deficiency and delinquency (Stewart, 2011). As well as a focus on psychopathology, including an emphasis on the familial origins of child behaviour problems, this period is also marked by a shift in focus in child welfare from the child to the parent, and the role of the voluntary sector in advancing services such as child guidance (Burchell, 2019). Here the role of parenting, interpersonal relationships and family dysfunction took centre stage, and issues such as 'maladjustment' and 'truancy' were perceived as outward manifestations of inner psychological processes (Black 1983; Judkins, 1948).

Although very separate disciplines, it could be argued that child psychiatry, safeguarding and child protection are to an extent intertwined. For example, the appointment of the first psychiatric social worker, in 1912 in the USA, was influenced by Freud's theories and a growing concern about the 'proper handling of delinquents' (Alexander, 1972; Brenner, 1974; Huff, 1998). Further influenced by psychiatrist Adolf Meyer's biographical approach to childhood problems, the role of the psychiatric social worker was to prepare a 'social history' of the child (with a focus on family background, health, interests, education, etc.) (Lamb, 2016). In the child guidance clinics, professionals from different disciplines – child psychiatrists, psychologists and social workers – worked together, with the child psychiatrist perceived as the leading discipline. With the aid of psychological tests and social work reports, it was the psychiatrist's role to identify the underlying causes of the maladjustment and to develop treatment, from play therapy and psychotherapy through to individual remedial teaching and family therapy (Sampson, 1976).

This was, in short, a medicalised approach to psychological and emotional problems in childhood, based on a form of medical holism (Stewart, 2009). All disciplines catered (and cater) for children with complex mental health needs (Black, 1983). Nevertheless, it should be acknowledged that social work and psychology/psychiatry grew from different origins: the first can be seen as the product of the child rescue movement and philanthropy, whereas the latter is associated with the biomedical and, later, the psychodynamic model (Burchell, 2019; Hall, 2007). As such, at a time when child philanthropy developed with a focus on supporting neglected and vulnerable children, child psychiatry started to develop with a focus on (biological, early trauma) causal factors in abnormal development in childhood and child psychopathology (Stewart, 2009, 2011).

The concept of 'development' links the biological facts of immaturity with the social aspect of childhood (e.g. see Gesell's work), i.e. the role of the family, and is reflected in psychological and sociological approaches, as well as the socio-political context of childhood (Cowie, 2019; Weizmann & Harris, 2012). In the first half of the 20th century, new social work and psychodynamic influences (e.g. work by Freud and Fairbairn) started to draw further attention to the quality of family relationships. Scottish psychiatrist and psychoanalyst W.R.D. (Ronald) Fairbairn popularised the term 'object relations' (the relationship between child and significant other), presenting this as the prototype for later expectations and experiences regarding relationships, and has affected child welfare practice in both the United Kingdom and the United States (Fuller, 1985; Raines, 2014). Unlike Freud, the founder of psychoanalysis and the theory of psychosexual development, Fairbairn did not believe that the libido was primarily aimed at pleasure, but instead at making relationships with objects external to the self (Bliss, 2010).

This marked a shift in practice, with a particular focus on the mother–child relationship and maternal inadequacies, taken further by British psychiatrist John Bowlby's theory of attachment (1988, 1998). With his theory, Bowlby emphasised and to an extent – with support from developmental psychologist Mary Ainsworth's strange situation experiment – also evidenced the importance of a secure and trusting mother–infant bond to the development and mental health of the child (Ainsworth et al., 2015; Bowlby, 1998). Some would however argue that Bowlby's idea of a naturally given maternal bond readily served to reinforce traditional gender roles in post-WWII Britain, as well as helping prevent the feminisation of the workplace (Polat, 2016; Riley, 1983). Others would argue that the experiences of early life have a lasting legacy, and that attachment theory has illuminated this field and deepened the understanding of educators (e.g. through nurture groups in schools) and child psychotherapists/counsellors, e.g. where children's attachment relationships have been disrupted through separation and loss (Cowie, 2019; Mesman et al., 2016). The development of social services and mental health support following the Second World War will be discussed further in the next section.

1.4 The NHS, the welfare state and social services: an improvement?

The institutions of Britain's welfare state were consolidated in the aftermath of the Second World War, coinciding with the establishment of the National Health Service (NHS) in 1948. The NHS appeared at a time when health care was seen as a crucial solution to solving, as the social reformer William Beveridge declared, one of the 'five giants' – want, disease, squalor, ignorance and idleness (Abel-Smith, 1992; Whiteside, 2014). The main position here was that health care should be a right, and not something bestowed erratically via charity, and was stimulated by the perception that 'there was a better way of doing things'. The key principles of the NHS were eligibility and free care, financed almost entirely from central taxation (Mossialos et al., 2000). The rapid improvements in population health that the NHS brought about caused a significant increase in life expectancy; but in turn this caused social care to be required for longer. Social care, social welfare and social work are often used in the same breath; and, as with the child rescue movement, they involve and incorporate informal networks of support and assistance as well as service funding following assessments by social work and other professions (Cylus et al., 2018; Dixon & Mossialos, 2002).

The provision of social care by local councils did not change when the NHS was created. The child guidance clinics continued to exist for a period of time, although they had been incorporated into the welfare state after the Second World War (Stewart, 2009, 2011). The welfare state added an additional concept to the understanding and perception of childhood and related wellbeing and safeguarding needs, namely the notion of the child as a 'public responsibility', influenced by the report of the Care of Children Committee, chaired by Myra Curtis, on child care and children's homes, which preceded and influenced the Children's Act of 1948 (Care of Children Committee, 1946; Hendrick, 1997; Lynch, 2019). The report described/discussed the state of affairs in children's homes in terms of utter loneliness, devoid of 'anyone to whom he [the child] could turn who was vitally interested in his welfare or who cared from him as a person'. This is interesting in light of research that highlights the caring nature of children's homes and institutions. For example Moss et al. (2017) researched child welfare and emigration institutions in 1870–1914, and argue that the image of uncaring and emotionally distant institutions does not reflect the ideology and practice of these (philanthropic) societies.

The last 150 years has seen numerous changes and policy initiatives concerning children's services: e.g. the establishment of the Charity Organisation Society in 1869, introducing a system of personal social work; the founding of the National Society for the Prevention of Cruelty to Children (NSPCC) in 1884; and the enactment of the Prevention of Cruelty to, and Protection of, Children Act 1889 (the Children's Charter). These were instigated by various and differing catalysts, some known and some unknown. For example, the Royal Society for the Prevention of Cruelty to Animals (RSPCA) was established in 1824, well before the NSPCC (Flegel, 2006). It was through the forum of the RSPCA and its American counterpart, the American Society for the Prevention of Cruelty to Animals (ASPCA), that the first child cruelty cases were successfully brought to court (Creighton, 1993; Markel, 2009).

The NSPCC originated as the London Society for the Prevention of Cruelty to Children (London SPCC) in 1884. After five years of campaigning by the London SPCC, in 1889 Parliament passed the first ever UK law to protect children from abuse and neglect. By then there were branches across the UK, so it was renamed the National Society in 1889 (NSPCC, 2019). More recently, the 1980s saw a rise in child sexual abuse reports and increased public concern about the way this was dealt with, culminating in the publication of the United Nations Convention on the Rights of the Child (UNCRC) in 1989. This marked a key turning point, highlighting the need for agencies to work together in meeting the needs of children (Cottrell & Kraam, 2005). When it comes to child safeguarding, protection and mental health support, there continues to be a complex mix of teams involved, with evidence of poor integration of welfare, mental health services and social care (Action for Children et al., 2018; Frost et al., 2005; Priest et al., 2011).

Since the inception of the child guidance clinics, there have been numerous developments around child psychiatry, child abuse and neglect. These include the establishment of a number of Acts in the UK (e.g. the Children Act 1948, which abolished the ad hoc arrangements for children in care, and the Children and Families Act 2014, with a focus on greater protection for vulnerable children), as well as the establishment of the Child and Adolescent Mental Health Services (CAMHS) in the 1990s (Bentley et al., 2016; Cottrell & Kraam, 2005).

Yet, the effectiveness of individual professions is open to debate, as is evident from the numerous reviews undertaken in the UK in relation to children's services – such as by Lord Laming (2009) and Professor Eileen Munro (2011) – highlighting a need for agencies and professionals to work together. For example, the Laming enquiry reports on the circumstances surrounding the horrific death of Victoria Climbié at the hands of her aunt and the aunt's boyfriend. The findings highlighted failings in individual practice, as well as poor inter-agency working and a failure of senior managers in various organisations to take responsibility for failings (Balen & Masson, 2007). At the same time, the Munro review of child protection highlights a need for conditions that enable professionals to make the best judgements about the help to give to children, young people and families.

In 2012 the most wide-ranging reforms to the NHS since it was founded in 1948 were introduced through the Health and Social Care Act, giving individual councils in England responsibility for improving the health of their populations (Peckham et al., 2015). Public health teams were transferred from the NHS to local authorities (LAs), accompanied by a ring-fenced public health grant (Jehu et al., 2018). Yet, balanced against competing demands for financial resources, democratic leverage and ongoing cuts to services, in many cases resources do not end up where they are most needed, such as in child safeguarding, protection and mental health support. Thus, issues around multidisciplinary teamwork between the different teams and professions (social workers, psychologists, psychiatrists and educationalists) and ongoing cuts to funding to services for the most vulnerable children continue to disadvantage certain families and children (Frost et al., 2017; Höjer et al., 2017; Jackson & Höjer, 2013).

Moreover, it could be argued that the notion of 'deservedness' has fed into the creation of the welfare state functioning as an insurance-based system, with a clear relationship between paying your dues and deserving help. For example, there is evidence of age, socio-economic and ethnic inequality in NHS provision (Shah & Cook, 2008). Over the years various economic crises have mounted sustained attacks on collective welfare, introducing charges and market criteria into these (Sales, 2002). Currently, traditional goals of social justice and collective responsibility for public services have been abandoned in favour of individual achievement and neoliberalism. This also means that young people have to seek out pathways to resilience (the ability to overcome adversity) and take advantage of whatever opportunities and resources are available to them (Sims-Schouten & Edwards, 2016). As such, so-called 'disordered' or 'delinquent' behaviours in 'troubled' young people may actually signify pathways to hidden resilience that, just like the ones adopted by their 'well-behaved' peers, are simply focused on the need to create powerful and influential identities for themselves (Ungar, 2002, 2004, 2005). Yet, there is evidence of an increased cultur-alisation as the stimulus for entitlement and access to support, thereby creating new stratifications of exclusion and inclusion (Jørgensen & Thomsen, 2018). This focus on individual accountability, responsibility and eligibility strongly resembles the 'deserving/undeserving' criteria introduced by the Poor Law of 1834.

1.5 The deserving/undeserving paradigm through time

A coordinated strategy for safeguarding and mental health provision in childhood was not formulated until the second half of the 20th century. Until then, and influenced by a range of approaches – from older tra-ditions of morality (influenced by the child rescue movement), 'common-sense' or 'deservedness' to psychoanalytic influences (Freud, Fairbairn and later Bowlby's attachment theory) – child welfare and mental health practices were disorganised (Cradock, 2014; Delap, 2015; Hacking, 1991; Raines, 2014). This resulted in a patchwork of practices, with the testimony of children from 'respectable' homes more likely to be heard than those from 'bad' or 'wretched' backgrounds. In this section I will show how the 'deserving/undeserving' paradigm is ingrained in past and present conceptions regarding safeguarding and mental health in childhood.

Both currently and in the past there is evidence of children and families missing out on support and intervention due to their complex needs, budget cuts and ever-changing thresholds (e.g. see Fong et al., 2018; Morrison, 2016; Rivett & Kelly, 2006). Here, there is a tendency to ignore underlying causal factors and generative mechanisms (e.g. material and institutional factors such as financial cuts and failures in multidisciplinary teamwork) in favour of a focus on deservedness/ undeservedness. An example of this is the response of agencies and professionals (e.g. policy and social services) in relation to the sexual exploitation scandals in various cities in the UK (Rotherham, Derby, Oxford and elsewhere) where girls as young as 13 years old were abused and described as 'out of control', 'streetwise' and 'akin to prostitutes' (Delap, 2015; Ellis, 2020; Morrison, 2016; Sims-Schouten et al., 2019). This strongly resembles 'The Maiden Tribute of Modern

Babylon', W.T. Stead's exposure of child prostitution in London, published in the *Pall Mall Gazette*, alluding to a need for more support and awareness regarding child protection and care (Stead, 1885). Current neoliberal practices with a focus on individual behaviour and self-responsibility can be traced back to practices enforced by the Charity Organisation Society, which worked with the Poor Law authorities in developing a system of personal social work grounded in 'deservedness' (Skinner & Thomas, 2018).

Notions to do with the 'psychosocial', 'wellbeing', 'morality' and 'behaviour' are highly influential in past and present conceptualisations of safeguarding and mental health support in childhood, and are often used to refer to a relationship of mind, body and social environment (Fong et al., 2018; Jones et al., 2018; Sohasky, 2015). The focus here is largely on a reductionist or isolated notion of the individual, who is blamed for their 'bad' behaviour, rather than on large-scale social structures (Dagnan, 2007; Toms, 2012). In practice this translates to assessments and interventions at various levels, from individual experiences and behaviour through to dynamics in the immediate social context, essentially locating 'problems' (mental health issues, abuse and neglect) in the family (Chettiar, 2012; Singh & Tuomainen, 2015; Slack & Webber, 2008). This positioning of the family as a crucial mediating point between the individual and the larger society has been influenced by the child rescue movement, as well as the wider medical, psychological, sociological and historical disciplines. For example, Bowlby (1988) emphasised the emotional dynamics of the mother–child relationship as a crucial factor in infant mental health and wellbeing, comparing mother-love to vitamins for physical health (see also Tasca et al., 2012). At the same time, sociologist/social politicist Richard Titmuss argued that the way in which children are socialised within families is of critical importance to the 'health' of societies, and that it is the family that is the 'central mechanism' for the transmission of culture (Chettiar, 2012; Welshman, 2004).

What current and past ideologies and related practices regarding safeguarding and mental health in childhood have in common is a location of problems in the family (e.g. through the construction of 'problematic families' and more recently the controversial 'troubled families' programme, launched in 2012) and the child (the fact that some children have immoral tendencies, either by nature or as a function of parental issues, such as alcoholism) (Delap, 2015; Sims-Schouten et al., 2019). Other approaches focus on the influence of adverse experiences in childhood (ACEs), highlighting that it is the child's (family) environment, and not the child, that is to blame for vulnerability and (negative) health and wellbeing behaviours (Hughes et al., 2016). Nevertheless, notions of morality and the ability to distinguish between choosing good and evil, and related behaviour, was a concern of psychiatrists and physicians (such as Rush, James Cowles Prichard, Emil Kraepelin and Maudsley) in the 19th and early 20th centuries, and confusion caused by unclear terms persists today (Horley, 2014).

There is evidence that children admitted to the asylum in the 19th century were admitted for much the same reasons as children are admitted to psychiatric wards today: they were unmanageable in the community or in the institutions from which they were referred (Sims-Schouten et al., 2019; Skinner & Thomas, 2018; Sohasky, 2015). Yet, this consistent focus on 'child rescue' through intervention/prevention problematically directs attention away from structural explanation, including political and economic causes (Moss et al, 2017). By putting the 'blame' and onus on families, structural and political causes of these patterns were (and still are) too easily dismissed. Moreover, there is evidence that certain children and families consistently miss out on the support they so desperately need. For example, both during the period of the child rescue movement and in contemporary society there is evidence of cutbacks on resources to support vulnerable children and families (Action for Children et al., 2018; Schene, 1998; Sims-Schouten et al., 2019). Additionally, both in past and current times children were and are categorised in terms of 'well-behaved/badly behaved' or 'clean-minded' and 'foul-minded', with often little recognition of the fact that institutional environments might also be sites of abuse. Think for example about the abuse stories and reports linked to various child migration schemes, such as the Canadian British Home Child movement (1869–1932) and the Australian Child Migration scheme (1940–1970) (Constantine, 2013; Lynch, 2015; Morton, 2014). Yet, stories of institutional child abuse are not just stories of the past – they happen time and time again.

Conclusion

Although the Poor Law of 1834 has been replaced by the modern welfare state in the UK, there is evidence that the 'deserving/undeserving' paradigm has lasting impact (Skinner & Thomas, 2018). Cuts to funding, high caseloads and poor integration of welfare, mental health services and social care mean that thresholds for care and support are constantly adjusted; and children get harmed in the process due to ever-increasing waiting times and slipping through the system (Rivett

& Kelly, 2006; Turner et al., 2015). Stigma also plays a significant role, and understandings are subject to the interests and values of the people and institutions attempting to define and interpret terms. Underlying causal factors (material, institutional and personal) are all too often ignored here in favour of a focus on 'deservedness'.

This book focuses on and centralises the group of young people referred to by Stein (2006) as 'victims', a term used for the most disadvantaged children who have spent time in care, have complex needs and have had the most damaging pre-care family experiences. Their time in care is characterised by further difficulties, instability and disruption; after leaving care they are likely to be unemployed and to become homeless, to be lonely and isolated and have mental health problems (Hood, 2016; Stein, 2006). It is this group of children, I argue, who often fall into the 'undeserving' category – when resources are scarce and judgements are made based on stigma, bias, which includes the notion that some children may be perceived as not fitting the 'right' criteria for support or that their needs are outside the remit of the various different agencies.

It should, however, also be acknowledged that the complexity of definitions, conceptualisations and understandings of childhood – where some focus on the 'innocence of the child' and others view the child as an active agent in the perpetuation of pauperism through truancy and 'bad' behaviour – means there is no neat fit between childhood and the 'deserving/undeserving' paradigm (Morton, 2014). As such, the developing status of childhood and the place of children within society also need to be viewed and acknowledged in light of this (Prout & James, 1997). Whilst some argue that the 20th and 21st are the 'centuries of the child', others (e.g. Pollock, 1983) take issue with the suggestion that children were treated as 'mini adults' in historic times, arguing that all centuries (to an extent) have taken account of the different phase that is childhood. Moreover, definitions and interpretations of 'childhood' also vary according to context, such as in legal terms (e.g. see the NSPCC website): in most situations a 'child' is someone who is under 18, whilst in some contexts, such as children's hearings and child protection orders, a child is defined as a person under 16 years of age. Thus, there is a need to shed light on contextual factors and causal mechanisms and processes that impact on how people make sense of safeguarding and mental health in childhood. This will be further discussed and explored in the next chapter, which introduces the critical realist ontology that forms the basis for the research and analysis of data presented in this book.

References

Abel-Smith, Brian (1992). The Beveridge report: its origins and outcomes. *International Social Security Review*, 45(1–2), 5–16. doi:10.1111/j.1468-1246X. 1992.tb00900.x.

Action for Children, NCB, The Children's Society, NSPCC and Barnardo's (2018). Children and Young people's services, funding and spending 2010/ 2011 to 2017/2018. https://www.childrenssociety.org.uk/sites/default/files/ childrens-services-funding-csfa-briefing_final.pdf.

Ainsworth, M.D.S., Blehar, M.C., Waters, E. and Wall, S.N. (2015). *Patterns of Attachment: A Psychological Study of the Strange Situation.* Hove: Psychology Press.

Alexander, L.B. (1972). Social work's Freudian deluge: myth or reality? *Social Service Review*, 46(4), 517–538.

Andrews, A., Briggs, A., Porter, R., Tucker, P. and Waddington, K. (1997). *The History of Bethlem.* London and New York: Routledge.

Anon. (2017). As a charity boss, I despair of Victorian attitudes ruining our good work. *Guardian*, 28 February. https://www.theguardian.com/volunta ry-sector-network/2017/feb/28/charity-boss-despair-victorian-a ttitudes-ruining-good-work.

Arnold, C. (2008). *Bedlam: London and Its Mad.* London: Pocket Books.

Atherton, M. (2011). Deserving of charity or deserving of better? The continuing legacy of the 1834 Poor Law Amendment Act for Britain's deaf population. *Review of Disability Studies*, 7(3–4), 18–25.

Balen, R. and Masson, H. (2007). The Victoria Climbié case: social work education for practice in children and families' work before and since. *Child & Family Social Work*, 13(2), 121–132.

Bentley, H., O'Hagan, O, Raff, A. and Bhatti, I. (2016). *How Safe Are Our Children? The Most Comprehensive Overview of Child Protection in the UK.* London: NSPCC. https://learning.nspcc.org.uk/media/1359/how-safe-children-2016-report.pdf.

Bergland, C. (2017). The neuroscience of contagious laughter. *Psychology Today*, 29 September. https://www.psychologytoday.com/gb/blog/the-athletes-way/201709/the-neuroscience-contagious-laughter.

Black, N. (1983). Are child guidance clinics an anachronism? *Archives of Disease in Childhood*, 58, 644–645.

Bliss, S. (2010). The 'internal saboteur': contributions of W.R.D. Fairbairn in understanding and treating self-harming adolescents. *Journal of Social Work Practice*, 24(2), 227–237. doi:10.1080/02650531003741744.

Bowlby, J. (1988). *A Secure Base: Parent-Child Attachment and Healthy Human Development.* London: Routledge.

Bowlby, J. (1998). *Attachment and Loss* (Vol. 3). London: Random House.

Brenner, C. (1974). *An Elementary Textbook of Psychoanalysis.* New York: Anchor.

Burchell, A. (2019). At the margins of the medical? Educational psychology, child guidance and therapy in provincial England, c.1945–1974. *Social History of Medicine*, hkz097. doi:10.1093/shm/hkz097.

Campbell, D. (2017). Thousands of mental health patients spend years on secure wards. *Guardian*, 20 July. https://www.theguardian.com/society/2017/jul/20/thousands-of-mental-health-patients-spend-years-on-secure-wards-nhs.

Care of Children Committee (1946). *Report of the Care of Children Committee*. London: HMSO.

Carter, P., James, J. and King, S.A. (2019). Punishing paupers? Control, discipline and mental health in the Southwell Workhouse, 1836–1871. *Rural History*, 30, 161–180.

Chettiar, T. (2012). Democratizing mental health: motherhood, therapeutic community and the emergence of the psychiatric family at the Cassel Hospital in post-Second World War Britain. *History of the Human Sciences*, 25(5), 107–122.

Constantine, S. (2013). *Empire, Migration and Identity in the British World*. Manchester: Manchester University Press.

Cottrell, D. and Kraam, A. (2005). Growing up? A history of CAMHS (1987–2005). *Child and Adolescent Mental Health*, 10(3), 111–117.

Cowie, H. (2019). *From Birth to Sixteen: Children's Health, Social, Emotional and Linguistic Development*. London: Routledge.

Cox, P. (2013). *Bad Girls in Britain: Gender, Justice and Welfare, 1900–1950*. Basingstoke: Palgrave Macmillan.

Cradock, G. (2014). Who owns child abuse? *Social Sciences*, 3, 854–870.

Creighton, S.J. (1993). Organized abuse: the NSPCC experience. *Child Abuse Review*, 2(4), 232–242.

Croll, A. (2017). Reconciled gradually to the system of indoor relief: the Poor Law in Wales during the 'crusade against out-relief', c.1870–c.1890. *Family & Community History*, 20, 121–144.

Cromby, J. and Harper, D.J. (2009). Paranoia: A social account. *Theory & Psychology*, 19(3), 335–361. doi:10.1177/0959354309104158.

Cylus, J., Roland, D., Nolte, E., Corbett, J., Jones, K., Forder, J. and Sussex, J. (2018). Identifying options for funding the NHS and social care in the UK: international evidence. Health Foundation Working Paper 3.

Dagnan, D. (2007). Psychosocial intervention for people with learning disabilities. *Advances in Mental Health and Learning Disabilities* 1(2), 3–7.

DeGarmo, J. (2015). We are failing our children. *HuffPost*, 7 August. https://www.huffpost.com/entry/we-are-failing-our-childr_b_7945172.

Delap, L. (2015). Child welfare, child protection and sexual abuse, 1918–1990, *History & Policy*. http://www.historyandpolicy.org/policy-papers/papers/child-welfare-child-protection-and-sexual-abuse-1918-1990.

Dixon, A. and Mossialos, E. (2002). Social insurance: not much to write home about? *Health Service Journal*, 112(5789), 24–26.

Dobbin, F. (1994). *Forging Industrial Policy: The United States, Britain, and France in the Railway Age*. New York: Cambridge University Press.

Ellis, K. (2020). Blame and culpability in children's narratives of sexual abuse. *Child Abuse Review*, 28(6), 405–417.

Flegel, M. (2006). Changing faces: the NSPCC and the use of photography in the construction of cruelty to children. *Victorian Periodicals Review*, 39(1), 1–20.

Fong, H.-F., Alegria, M., Bair-Merritt, M.H. and Beardslee, W. (2018). Factors associated with mental health services referrals for children investigated by child welfare. *Child Abuse & Neglect*, 79, 401–412. doi:10.1016/j.chiabu.2018.01.020.

Frost, E., Höjer, S., Campanini, A., Sicora, A. and Kullberg, K. (2017). Why do they stay? A study of resilient child protection workers in three European countries. *European Journal of Social Work*, 21(4), 485–497. doi:10.1080/13691457.2017.1291493.

Frost, N., Robinson, M. and Anning, A. (2005). Social workers in multidisciplinary teams: issues and dilemmas for professional practice. *Child & Family Social Work*, 10(3), 187–196.

Fuller, P. (1985). Introduction, in C. Rycroft, *Psychoanalysis and Beyond*, edited by P. Fuller. London: Chatto & Windus, 1–38.

Gatty, M. (Ed.) (1871). *Aunt Judy's Christmas Volume for Young People*. London: Bell and Daldy.

Gelfand, T. (1984). A 'monarchical profession' in the old regime: surgeons, ordinary practitioners, and medical professionalization in eighteenth-century France, in Geison, G.L. (Ed.), *Professions and the French State, 1700–1900*. Philadelphia: University of Pennsylvania Press), 149–180.

Gingell, K. (2001). The forgotten children: children admitted to a county asylum between 1854 and 1900. *Psychiatric Bulletin*, 25, 432–434.

Griesinger, W. (1867). *Mental Pathology and Therapeutics*. London: New Sydenham Society.

Groves, J. (2013). Now even claimants admit they are getting too much in benefits: 59 per cent of those given handouts think they discourage work. *Mail Online*, 4 September. https://www.dailymail.co.uk/news/article-2410622/Benefits-59-cent-given-handouts-think-discourage-work.html.

Hacking, I. (1991). The making and molding of child abuse. *Critical Inquiry*, 17(2), 253–288.

Hall, G. Stanley (1904). *Adolescence: Its Psychology and Its Relations to Physiology, Anthropology, Sociology, Sex, Crime, Religion and Education*. New York: Appleton.

Hall, J. (2007). The emergence of clinical psychology in Britain from 1943 to 1952. Part I: core tasks and the professionalisation process. *History & Philosophy of Psychology*, 9, 29–55.

Hendrick, H. (1994). *Child Welfare: England 1872–1989*. Routledge: London.

Hendrick, H. (1997). Constructions and reconstructions of British childhood: an interpretative survey, 1800 to the present. In: James, A. and Prout, A. (Eds.), *Constructing and Reconstructing Childhood*. London: Routledge, 34–62.

Higginbotham, P. (2017). *Children's Homes. A History of Institutional Care for Britain's Young*. Barnsley: Pen & Sword History.

Höjer, S., Frost, L., Campanini, A., Sicora, A. and Kullberg, K. (2017). Outsiders and learners: negotiating meaning in comparative European social work research practice. *Qualitative Social Work*, 16(4), 465–480. doi:10.1177/1473325015621124.

Hood, R. (2016). How professionals talk about complex cases: a critical discourse analysis. *Child & Family Social Work*, 21(2), 125–135. doi:10.1111/cfs.12122.

Horley, J. (2014). The emergence and development of psychopathy. *History of the Human Sciences*, 27(5), 91–110.

Huff, D. (1998). *Progress and Reform: An Illustrated History of Social Work 1860–1940*. Washington: National Association of Social Workers Press.

Huffadine, L. (2015). Is your toddler a psychopath? *Mail Online*, 11 September. https://www.dailymail.co.uk/news/article-3230167/Is-child-psychopath-Traits-lack-emotion-empathy-detected-just-THREE-years-old.html.

Hughes, K., Lowey, H., Quigg, Z. and Bellis, M.A. (2016). Relationships between adverse childhood experiences and adult mental well-being: results from an English national household survey. *BMC Public Health*, 16, art. 222. doi:10.1186/s12889-016-2906-3.

Hurren, E. (2015). *Protesting about Pauperism, Poverty, Politics and Poor Relief in Late-Victorian England 1870–1900*. Woodbridge: Royal Historical Society.

Khan, J. (2012). Can you call a 9-year-old a psychopath? *New York Times*, 11 May. https://www.nytimes.com/2012/05/13/magazine/can-you-call-a-9-year-old-a-psychopath.html.

Jackson, S. and Höjer, I. (2013). Prioritising education for children looked after away from home. *European Journal of Social Work*, 16(1), 1–5. doi:10.1080/13691457.2012.763108.

Jehu, L.M., Visram, S., Marks, L., Hunter, D.J., Davis, H., Mason, A., Lui, D. and Smithson, J. (2018). Directors of public health as 'a protected species': qualitative study of the changing role of public health professionals in England following the 2013 reforms. *Journal of Public Health*, 40(3), 203–210.

Jones, T.M., Nurius, P., Song, C. and Fleming, C.M. (2018). Modeling life course pathways from adverse childhood experiences to adult mental health. *Child Abuse & Neglect*, 80, 32–40. doi:10.1016/j.chiabu.2018.03.005.

Jørgensen, M.B. and Thomsen, T.L. (2018). 'Needed but undeserving': contestations of entitlement in the Danish policy framework on migration and integration. In: Fossum, J., Kastoryano, R. and Siim, B. (Eds.), *Diversity and Contestations over Nationalism in Europe and Canada*. London: Palgrave Macmillan, 337–364.

Judkins, B. (1948). Adoptive parents in a child guidance clinic. *American Journal of Orthopsychiatry, Mental Health & Social Justice*, 18(2), 257–264. doi:10.1111/j.1939-0025.1948.tb05083.x.

Keane, A.M. (1987). *Mental Health Policy in Scotland,1908–1960*. PhD thesis, University of Edinburgh. file:///C:/Users/Wendy/AppData/Local/Temp/381871.pdf.

King, S. (2003). Making the most of opportunity: the economy of makeshifts in the early modern north. In: S. King and A. Tomkins (Eds.), *The Poor in England 1700–1850: An Economy of Makeshifts*. Manchester and New York: Manchester University Press, 228–257.

King, S. (2018). *Sickness, Medical Welfare and the English Poor, 1750–1834*. Manchester: Manchester University Press.

King, S. (2019). *Writing the Lives of the English Poor, 1750s–1830s*. Montreal and Kingston: McGill-Queen's University Press.

Lamb, S. (2016). 'My resisting getting well': neurasthenia and subconscious conflict in patient–psychiatrist interactions in prewar America. *Journal of the History of Behavioural Sciences*, 52(2), 124–145.

Laming, Lord (2009). *The Protection of Children in England: A Progress Report*. London: The Stationery Office, https://assets.publishing.service.gov. uk/government/uploads/system/uploads/attachment_data/file/328117/The_ Protection_of_Children_in_England.pdf.

Lynch, G. (2015). *Remembering Child Migration: Faith, Nation-Building and Wounds of Charity*. London: Bloomsbury.

Lynch, G. (2019). Pathways to the 1946 Curtis Report and the post-war reconstruction of children's out-of-home care. *Contemporary British History*, 34(1), 22–43.

MacKinnon, M. (1987). English Poor Law policy and the crusade against outdoor relief. *Journal of Economic History*, 47(3), 603–625.

Markel, H. (2009). Case shined first light on abuse of children. *New York Times*, 14 December 2009. https://www.nytimes.com/2009/12/15/health/15abus. html.

Mash, E. and Wolfe, D. (2019). *Abnormal Child Psychology*. Belmont, CA: Wadsworth.

Maudsley, H. (1879), *The Pathology of Mind*. London: Macmillan.

Mayhew, H. (1968). *London Labour and the London Poor* (Vol. 1). New York: Dover.

Mayhew, H. (2008). *London Labour and the London Poor: A Selection by Rosemary O'Day and David England*. Ware: Wordsworth Editions.

Mayhew, H. (2010). *London Labour and the London Poor*, edited by R. Douglas-Fairhurst. Oxford: Oxford University Press.

Melling, J., Adair, R. and Forsythe, B. (1997). 'A proper lunatic for two years': pauper lunatic children in Victorian and Edwardian England. Child admissions to the Devon County Asylum, 1845–1914, *Journal of Social History*, 31(2), 371–394.

Mesman, J., van Ijzendoorn, M.H. and Sagi-Schwartz, A. (2016). Cross-cultural patterns of attachment: universal and contextual dimensions. In: J. Cassidy and P. Shaver (Eds.), *Handbook of Attachment: Theory, Research, and Clinical Applications* (3rd edn). New York: Guilford Press, 852–877.

Morrison, J. (2016). *Familiar Strangers, Juvenile Panics and the British Press: The Decline of Social Trust*. London: Palgrave Macmillan.

Morton, S. (2014). *Wisdom, Justice, Charity: Canadian Social Welfare through the Life of Jane B. Wisdom, 1884–1975*. Toronto: University of Toronto Press.

Moruzi, K. (2017). 'Donations need not be large to be acceptable': children, charity and the Great Ormond Street Children's Hospital in Aunt Judy's Magazine, 1868–1885. *Victorian Periodicals Review*, 50(1), 190–213.

Moss, E., Wildman, C., Lamont, R. and Kelly, L. (2017). Rethinking child welfare and emigration institutions, 1870–1914. *Cultural and Social History*, 14(5), 647–668.

Mossialos, E., Dixon, A. and McKee, M. (2000). Paying for the NHS: first decide how much we are willing to pay, then think about how to collect it. *British Medical Journal*, 320(7229), 197–198.

Münch, O. (2018). Henry Mayhew and the street traders of Victorian London: a cultural exchange with material consequences. *London Journal*, 43(1), 53–71. doi:10.1080/03058034.2017.1333761.

Munro, E. (2011). *The Munro Report of Child Protection: Final Report. A Child-Centred System*. London: The Stationery Office.

NSPCC (2019). A history of child protection in the UK. https://learning.nspcc. org.uk/child-protection-system/history-of-child-protection-in-the-uk.

Parry-Jones, W.L. (1972). *The Trade in Lunacy: A Study of Private Madhouses in England in the Eighteenth and Nineteenth Centuries*. London: Routledge & Kegan Paul.

Partridge, G.E. (1912). *Genetic Philosophy of Education: An Epitome of the Published Writings of G. Stanley Hall*. New York: New International Encyclopedia.

Peckham, S., Falconer, J., Gillam, S. et al. (2015). The organisation and delivery of health improvement in general practice and primary care: a scoping study. *Health Services and Delivery Research*, 3(29). Southampton (UK): NIHR Journals Library. doi:10.3310/hsdr03290.

Polat, B. (2016). Before attachment theory: separation research at the Tavistock Clinic, 1948–1956. *Journal of the History of Behavioral Sciences*, 53(1), 48–70.

Pollock, L. (1983). *Forgotten Children: Parent–Child Relations from 1500 to 1900*. Cambridge: Cambridge University Press.

Price, K. (2012). 'Where is the fault?': The starvation of Edward Cooper at the Isle of Wight workhouse in 1877. *Social History of Medicine*, 26, 21–37.

Priest, P., Dunn, C., Hackett, J. and Wills, K. (2011). How can mental health professionals best be supported in working with people who experience significant stress? *Journal of Mental Health*, 20(6), 543–554.

Prout, A. and James, A. (1997). A new paradigm for the sociology of childhood? Provenance, promise and problems. In: A. James and A. Prout (Eds.), *Constructing and Reconstructing Childhood*. London: Routledge, 7–33.

Raines, W.C. (2014). Fairbairn's object relations theory and social work in child welfare. In: G.S. Clarke and D.E. Scharf (Eds.), *Fairbairn and the Object Relations Tradition*. London: Routledge.

Rauch, A. (1997). Parables and parodies: Margaret Gatty's audiences in the parables from nature. *Children's Literature*, 25, 138–150.

Rey, J.M., Assumpção, F.B., Bernad, C.A., Çuhadaroğlu, F.C., Evans, B., Fung, D., Harper, G., Loidreau, L., Ono, Y., Pūras, D., Remschmidt, H., Robertson, B., Rusakoskaya, O.A. and Schleimer, K. (2015). History of child and adolescent psychiatry. In: Rey, J.M (Ed.), *IACAPAP e-Textbook of Child and Adolescent Mental Health*. Geneva: International Association for Child and Adolescent Psychiatry and Allied Professions, 1–67.

Riley, D. (1983). *War in the Nursery*. London: Virago.

Rivett, M. and Kelly, S. (2006). 'From awareness to practice': children, domestic violence and child welfare. *Child Abuse Review*, 15(4), 224–242. doi:10.1002/car.945.

Roberts, D. (1963). How cruel was the Victorian Poor Law? *Historical Journal*, 6, 97–107.

Royden, M. (2017). *Tales from the 'Pool: A Collection of Liverpool Stories*. Liverpool: Creative Dreams.

Sales, R. (2002). The deserving and the undeserving? Refugees, asylum seekers and welfare in Britain. *Critical Social Policy*, 22(3), 456–478.

Sampson, O.C. (1976). Treatment practices in British child guidance clinics: an historical overview. *Educational Review*, 29(1), 13–29.

Schene, P.A. (1998). Past, present and future roles of child protective services. *Protecting Children from Abuse and Neglect*, 8(1), 23–38.

Shah, S.M. and Cook, D.G. (2008). Socio-economic determinants of casualty and NHS Direct use. *Journal of Public Health*, 30(1), 75–81.

Shore, H. (2003). Crime, criminal networks and the survival strategies of the poor in early eighteenth-century London. In: King, S. and Tomkins, A. (Eds.), *The Poor in England, 1700–1850: An Economy of Makeshifts*. Manchester and New York: Manchester University Press, 137–165.

Shuttleworth, G.E. (1903). On some slighter forms of mental defect in children and their treatment. *British Medical Journal*, 2(2231), 828–830.

Sims-Schouten, W. and Edwards, S. (2016). 'Man up!' Bullying and resilience within a neoliberal framework. *Journal of Youth Studies*, 19(10), 1382–1400.

Sims-Schouten, W., Skinner, A. and Rivett, K. (2019). Child safeguarding in light of the deserving/undeserving paradigm: a historical and contemporary analysis. *Child Abuse & Neglect*, 94. doi:10.1016/j.chiabu.2019.104025.

Singh, S.P. and Tuomainen, H. (2015). Transition from child to adult mental health services: needs, barriers, experiences and new models of care. *World Psychiatry*, 14(3), 358–361. doi:10.1002/wps.20266.

Skinner, A. and Thomas, N. (2018). 'A pest to society': the Charity Organisation Society's domiciliary assessments into the circumstances of poor families and children. *Children & Society*, 32, 133–144. doi:10.1111/chso.12237.

Slack, K. and Webber, M. (2008). Do we care? Adult mental health professionals' attitudes towards supporting service users' children, *Child & Family Social Work*, 13(1), 72–79.

Sohasky, K.E. (2015). Safeguarding the interests of the state from defective delinquent girls. *Journal of the History of Behavioral Sciences, 52*(1), 20–40. doi:10.1002/jhbs.21765.

Stead, W.T. (1885). *The Maiden Tribute of Modern Babylon*. London.

Stedman Jones, G. (1971). *Outcast London: A Study in the Relationship between Classes in Victorian Society*. Oxford: Clarendon.

Stein, M. (2006). Research review: young people leaving care. *Child and Family Social Work*, 11(3), 273–279.

Stewart, J. (2009). The scientific claims of British child guidance, 1918–45. *British Journal of the History of Science*, 45, 407–432.

Stewart, J. (2011). 'The dangerous age of childhood': child guidance and the 'normal' child in Great Britain, 1920–1950. *Paedagogica Historica*, 47, 785–803.

Strand, M. (2016). Historicizing social inequality: a Victorian archive for contemporary moral discourse. *American Journal of Cultural Sociology*, 5(1–2), 225–260.

Taithe, B. (Ed.) (1996). *The Essential Mayhew: Representing and Communicating the Poor*. London: Rivers Oram Press.

Tasca, C., Rapetti, M., Carta, M.G. and Fadda, B. (2012). Women and hysteria in the history of mental health. *Clinical Practice & Epidemiology in Mental Health*, 8, 110–119, doi:10.2174/1745017901208010110.

Taylor, S.J. (2015). Poverty, emigration and family: experiencing childhood poverty in late nineteenth-century Manchester. *Family & Community History*, 18, 91–103.

Taylor, S.J. (2016). *Child Insanity in England, 1845–1907*. Basingstoke: Palgrave Macmillan.

Thane, P. (2012). The 'big society' and the 'big state': creative tension or crowding out? *Twentieth Century British History*, 23, 408–429.

Toms, J. (2012). Political dimensions of 'the psychosocial': the 1948 International Congress on Mental Health and the Mental Hygiene Movement. *History of the Human Sciences*, 25(5), 91–106.

Turner, J., Hayward, R., Angel, K., Fulford, B., Hall, J., Millard, C. and Thomson, M. (2015). The history of mental health services in modern England: practitioner memories and the direction of future research. *Medical History*, 59(4), 599–624. doi:10.1017/mdh.2015.48.

Ungar, M. (2002). *Playing at Being Bad: The Hidden Resilience of Troubled Teens*. East Lawrencetown, NS: Pottersfield Press.

Ungar, M. (2004). *Nurturing Hidden Resilience in Troubled Youth*. Toronto: University of Toronto Press.

Ungar, M. (2005). *A Handbook for Working with Children and Youth: Pathways to Resilience across Cultures and Contexts*. Thousand Oaks, CA: Sage.

Ward, H. (1990). *The Charitable Relationship: Parents, Children and the Waifs and Strays Society*. PhD thesis, University of Bristol. https://research-information.bristol.ac.uk/files/34489504/292443.pdf.

Weizmann, F. and Harris, B. (2012). Arnold Gesell: The maturationist. In: Pickren, W.E., Dewsbury, D.A. and Wertheimer, M. (Eds.), *Portraits of Pioneers in Developmental Psychology*. New York: Psychology Press, 1–20.

Welshman, J. (2004). The unknown Titmuss, *Journal of Social Policy*, 33(2), 225–247.

Whiteside, N. (2014). The Beveridge Report and its implementation: a revolutionary project? *Histoire@Politique*, 3, 24–37.

Wilkins, R. (1987). Hallucinations in children and teenagers admitted to Bethlem Royal Hospital in the nineteenth century and their possible relevance to the incidence of schizophrenia. *Journal of Child Psychology and Psychiatry*, 28, 569–580.

2 Mental health and safeguarding through a critical realist lens

Given the development of safeguarding and mental health support practices in the UK and beyond, and the legacy of the deserving/undeserving paradigm therein (as discussed in Chapter 1), it is imperative that we study changes in institutions of social life, such as family and social care, within temporal (historiographical) contrasts. In this chapter I will show that, influenced by a range of conflicting ideologies, from medical naturalism to social constructionism, different professional groups adjudicate on the field of mental wellbeing with fundamental disagreement about thresholds and eligibility for support, dismissing historical and structural mechanisms. For example, historically the biomedical model of inheritance and determinism in relation to 'mental deficiency' encouraged the belief that some individuals were biologically degenerate without hope of reform (Pilgrim, 2014). Social constructionism, on the other hand, argues that our understanding of the world is produced in interaction, through social processes that are socio-historically contingent, without acknowledging that some problems, e.g. unemployment, stem from material and institutional conditions (Bhaskar, 1989; Patel & Pilgrim, 2018; Sims-Schouten et al., 2007; Sims-Schouten & Riley, 2014). The analytical framework adopted in this book draws on critical realism, a metatheory that uses elements from both social constructionist and biomedical models. Below I will explain (conflicting) ideologies that are currently adopted in research with a focus on mental illness and safeguarding, and explain why I feel that critical realist ontology provides a useful interface and way forward here.

2.1 Making sense of safeguarding needs and mental health problems in childhood: conflicting ideologies and epistemologies

Abuse, neglect and mental health issues in childhood might come to the attention of (child) psychiatrists/psychologists and social workers employed by local authorities, as well as general practitioners (GPs), teachers and youth workers, each with their own history, definitions and specialist epistemologies (Cradock, 2014; Pilgrim, 2014; Sims-Schouten et al., 2019). Child protective action and child mental health support are fundamentally political, and the different subfields and agencies can make it hard to follow up cases and establish best practice. It follows that research into safeguarding, abuse and mental health issues in childhood and related support needs to be viewed in light of dominant social-historical constructs and mechanisms, while simultaneously recognising that these constructs operate within a narrative of power and resistance (Hacking, 1991; Sohasky, 2015). Historical investigations can explain some of the mechanisms at play at the field level, influencing particular outcomes and practices (Mutch, 2014).

Social work in the UK is born from the 'child rescue' movement and has historically aligned itself with a pragmatic form of sociology. In practice this means that social work is marked by ongoing tension between a focus on social and personal empowerment on the one hand and social control and a disinclination to challenge existing social structures on the other (Houston, 2010). This tension can also be seen in the debate between structural social work and humanistic social work. Whilst humanistic social work originates from psychology and centralises social agency and self-actualisation, structural social work is a moral theory suggesting that social systems are intentionally designed to oppress marginalised populations (Carrillo, 2018; Mullaly, 1993; Payne, 2011). Modern child psychiatric services, on the other hand, have evolved from very different roots, and current practices are influenced by a range of (potentially conflicting) ideologies, from medical naturalism or biomedical approaches to social constructionist approaches (Cromby, 2016; Pilgrim, 2014; Roberts, 2014). Medical naturalism (or psychiatric positivism) is marked by the premise that mental illness simply exists 'out there', waiting to be verified by experts, whilst the epistemological assumption of social constructionism is that we can only know the world via the ways we represent it (Pilgrim, 2014). Whilst the biomedical approach to mental illness is restricted by a focus on diagnosis and deficits, also referred to as 'naive realism', social constructionist approaches are accused of putting too much focus on meaning-making at the expense of material and physiological factors (Sims-Schouten & Riley, 2018; Patel & Pilgrim, 2018). Neither provides a usable solution for practitioners (Pilgrim & Bentall, 1999).

The biomedical approach is limited by a belief in an immediate empirical reality treating mental illness as fundamentally pathological, emphasising pharmacological treatment to target presumed biological abnormalities (Deacon, 2013). Historically, biological determinants were used to explain deficiencies in those considered biologically degenerate and lacking mental capacity, encouraging the belief that such conditions were innate (Pilgrim, 2014) and linked to moral competence (Sohasky, 2015) – thus placing the responsibility with the individual. An example of this is 'feeblemindedness', a mental classification used in relation to heritability. Additionally, experts believed that intellectual deficiency generated moral incompetence, leading to delinquency and disordered behaviour (Melling et al., 1997; Taylor, 2016).

Social constructionism, on the other hand, argues that our understanding of the world is produced in interaction, through social processes that are socio-historically located, without acknowledging that some problems, e.g. unemployment, stem from material and institutional conditions (Bhaskar, 1989; Sims-Schouten & Riley, 2014). Social constructionist informed therapy (e.g. narrative therapy, social therapy, solution-focused brief therapy) and constructive therapy emphasise the importance of human relationships in wellbeing and development (Gergen, 2009; Mahoney & Granvold, 2005). In therapy mental health problems are treated as the by-product of troubled relations with others, with the therapist as participant-observer and participant-facilitator of the therapeutic conversation (McNamee & Gergen, 1992; White, 2011).

It follows that there is a need for an approach that brings together the range of epistemologies and ontologies of the varying disciplines. When it comes to safeguarding and mental health support in childhood, there includes a recognition and awareness of social structures and conditions that re-affirm or challenge systems of care, support, control and cure, including the day-to-day contradictions involving the 'personal' and 'political' (Fitzpatrick, 2005; Houston, 2010). Without this there is a danger that judgements are made on the basis of who is 'deserving' and 'undeserving' of support. Society is changing rapidly, and many child mental health specialists find themselves being forced to adopt society's agendas for 'disturbed' children (Gingell, 2001). Popular discourse around 'deservedness' – e.g. in relation to the vulnerability and/or malevolence of different types of children and their families – often acts as a locus for the manifestations of stigma, prejudices and deeper-seated anxiety, including perceptions of lifestyle choices, social-economic background and cultural characteristics (Morrison, 2016). Links are also made to social and economic factors that contributed to the 'respectability' of families and children.

Below I will outline critical realist ontology, and explain how this can be useful when making sense of practices and perceptions with a focus on safeguarding and mental health in childhood, drawing together different theoretical and philosophical frameworks.

2.2 Critical realism and mental health and safeguarding: a compromise?

Critical realism (CR) is an ontology associated with English philosopher (Ram) Roy Bhaskar (1989, 2014), and combines a general philosophy of science with a philosophy of social science to describe an interface between the natural and social worlds. As such, whilst proposing that there is an (objective) world that exists independently of people's perceptions, language and imagination, CR also recognises that part of that world consists of subjective interpretations that influence the way in which the world is perceived (O'Mahoney & Vincent, 2014). Here critical realism's main focus is to promote awareness as a central strategy for tackling inequality and uneven practices/perceptions, providing insight into the causal non-linear dynamics and generative mechanisms in the individual, the cultural sphere and wider society (Sims-Schouten et al., 2019). Critical realism's central premise is that the world is differentiated and stratified, and, in order to make sense of social life, we must engage with and understand the interplay between human agency (meaning-making, motivation, intentionality) and social structures (enduring patterns, social rules, norms and laws) (Fitzpatrick, 2005; Houston, 2010; Wilson, 2020). Within this, causal or generative powers are key, regarded as necessary tendencies of agents, social objects and structures that may or may not be activated, depending on conditions (Sayer, 2000). Critical realist informed stratified model of reality thus allows for the conceptualisation of the 'real' (exploring the causal mechanisms of events), the 'empirical' (experienced events) and the 'actual' (events and processes that occur) (Bhaskar, 2014; Sims-Schouten & Riley, 2014, 2018).

Taking safeguarding, child protection and mental health and wellbeing (from 1881 to the present) as a starting point, this means exploring:

- causal mechanisms that generate events, such as stress, trauma, as well as cuts to services (what Bhaskar calls the 'real' level);
- how those events are experienced by individuals, e.g. in relation to stigma (referred to by Bhaskar, 1989, 2014 as the empirical level), and

- events and processes in relation to child protection and mental health support currently in place or lacking (referred to by Bhaskar as the 'actual').

Critical realism does not claim to identify direct causal relationships between these factors; rather, it seeks to identify and explore how the real, empirical and actual may interact in complex, iterative ways that create the conditions of possibility for sense-making. When considering how people make sense of child abuse, neglect and mental health issues in childhood and related support, critical realism can therefore incorporate consideration of: material factors (e.g. income, socio-economic situation, budget cuts); institutional processes (e.g. the availability of support services and facilities); embodied mechanisms (e.g. stress, trauma); and discursive factors that may structure such sense-making.

Drawing on critical realism, it can be argued, for example, that parent wellbeing, as well as parenting skills and 'flaws', can be both a product of fatigue (e.g. Cooklin et al., 2012; Dunning & Giallo, 2012) and a product of societal expectations (e.g. Brady et al., 2015; Sims-Schouten & Riley, 2018). Similarly, a person's vulnerability and exposure to abuse and mental health risks can be attributed to a variety of interacting factors – such as hormones, inheritability, discourses of gender (which in turn impact on experiences of control, power, dominance), socioeconomic position and social status, as well as access to resources and treatment (Cromby, 2016; Sims-Schouten & Riley, 2018).

Thus, a critical realist ontology allows for the accommodation of material/embodied factors (e.g. hormonal imbalance, trauma) in relation to abuse, neglect and mental health problems in children, alongside a critical analysis of the way in which the respective concepts/issues/phenomena are described and conceptualised in society at a point in time (e.g. a critique of the interests served by psychiatric knowledge). CR's primacy of ontology forms the starting point here, whereas for positivists and social constructionists epistemology is primary (Bhaskar, 1989, 2014). Bhaskar draws attention to human agency, but also argues that intentionality (voluntary human action) does not simply construct social reality; and neither is human action itself mechanically determined by social reality. Instead, society exists prior to the lives of agents; but they become agents who reproduce or transform that society (Pilgrim & Bentall, 1999). This means taking account of the antecedent and current conditions that shape a person's experiences, as well as the fact that child abuse, neglect and mental health problems must be understood within its specific context of time and place – it is historically and geographically situated (see also

Mutch, 2014). As such, critical realism is instrumental in influencing the search for generative mechanisms, which might have combined to create a phenomenon over time, influencing particular outcomes and practices (Mutch, 2014).

Yet, whilst critical realism provides a crucial remedy to some of the pitfalls of employing either a social constructionist approach (extreme relativism) or a biomedical approach (naive realism), it has also received some criticism. One such criticism is that critical realism employs a dualist perspective in which causal mechanisms (i.e. non-discursive factors) are associated with 'closed' systems, while actual, concrete events operate in 'open' systems (Bhaskar, 2014; Scambler & Scambler, 2015). It could be argued that, partly in response to this, Bhaskar introduced the concept of 'dialectical critical realism', suggesting that causal mechanisms must be situated in a dialectically connected totality, which also includes within it historical processes and concrete events (Roberts, 2014; Scambler & Scambler, 2015). In line with this, Bhaskar (2014) refers to examples such as 'absence' (the fact that looking at what is missing in a social context or entity/institution/organisation will often provide insight into how that situation is going to or needs to change) and 'epistemological dialectic' (inconsistencies in cognitive or practical situations suggesting that something has been left out of the theoretical or practical mix). It is these issues that I contend are important when considering and examining safeguarding and mental health practices in childhood. In the next section I will take a closer look at generative mechanisms and causal factors that could play a role in practices and perceptions in relation to safeguarding and mental health in childhood.

2.3 Trauma, abuse, stigma and cuts to services as generative mechanisms

Drawing on Bhaskar's critical realist ontology (2014), I adopt a form of reasoning called retroduction, which involves moving from the level of observation and lived experiences to making (non-linear) inferences about underlying structures and mechanisms that may account for the phenomena involved. In this case this means that I am interested in the intersection between the material (e.g. income, socio-economic situation), institutional (e.g. the availability of support services and facilities), embodied (e.g. stress, trauma) and discursive factors, and how this may structure sense-making around abuse, neglect and mental health issues in childhood and related support (see also Sims-Schouten et al., 2019; Sims-Schouten & Riley, 2014).

Whilst material and institutional conditions represent events that are external to the person involved, embodiment encompasses the fact that conceptualisations/perceptions depend on and are interlinked with having a body with various sensorimotor capacities, and perception and action are fundamentally inseparable (Klin & Jones, 2007). As an example of embodiment, early experiences in relation to attachment and abuse/neglect and related trauma, as well as individual characteristics and hormonal imbalance, have all been associated with mental health problems and behavioural issues in childhood (Sims-Schouten & Hayden, 2017; Sims-Schouten & Riley, 2018). Yet, it is important to also locate this within the stratified non-linear dynamics of embodied experiences, material/institutional forces and social relationships that co-constitute subjectivity as well as having an ongoing influence on body–brain systems (Cromby & Harper, 2009).

As an example, irritability, anger or 'bad behaviour' could be a response to the perceived unreasonable actions of others or something due to low blood sugar and fatigue; but it could also be associated with chronic trauma (or a mix of factors) (e.g. Cooklin et al., 2012; Dunning & Giallo, 2012). Similarly, whilst the effect of hormones such as oestrogen (among other possible physiological causes) can be one route in accounting, for example, for the differing psychopathological profiles of men and women across the life span, other aspects relating to hegemonic masculinity (control, power, dominance), socio-economic position, roles, social status and access to resources and treatment are also critical in determining a person's vulnerability and exposure to mental health risks in society (Cromby & Harper, 2009; Pilgrim & Bentall, 1999; Sims-Schouten & Riley, 2018).

An example of this can be seen in a historical case file (Case 18451) from the Waifs and Strays Society, now known as the Children's Society. This involves a girl born in 1904 who is taken into care in 1914 due to an 'unsatisfactory home', which could refer to anything from parents neglecting the child through to alcohol abuse by one of the parents. The case file includes correspondence from a matron of a children's home, and education officer, a medical officer, the Union (Poor Law), a clergyman, Salvation Army authorities and the girl herself. Between 1914 and 1916 there is talk of 'good behaviour' as well as 'abnormal behaviour', which, according to the medical officer, can be linked to the fact that 'the girl has been criminally assaulted and that the appearances support the child's own story that the assaults have been of frequent occurrence'. Due to the 'peculiarity of her temperament' the children's home is, however, no longer able to look after her; at the same time (in 1921), it is made clear by the education officer that 'she is not a case to be dealt with under the Mental Deficiency Act'. After this (still in 1921), she is re-examined by the Medical Superintendent on account of her 'violent temper' and 'sullen, pert and rude behaviour' and 'inclination to quarrel with those around her'. As this behaviour normally only lasts a few days, the Medical Superintendent concludes that this is hormonal and something that 'synchronises with her menstrual periods'.

Drawing on critical realist ontology, it could be argued that in order to make sense of the mental health and safeguarding issues surrounding this young person, it is imperative to see this in light of the intersection between her embodied, material and institutional realities as causal and discursively mediated factors (i.e. the 'real' level), events and processes in relation to this (the 'actual'), and how this is experienced by her (the 'empirical').

Bhaskar's critical realism allows us to take account of the fact that notions to do with mental illness and 'keeping children safe' (i.e. safeguarding) are both socially constructed, as well as influenced by external factors and forces that can be real and independent of any one person or social group (Sayer, 2000). As an example of the latter, dissociative responding combined with extreme states of affect is often associated with those who have experienced trauma in the past (Leckman et al., 2007; Lysaker et al., 2011; Schalinski et al., 2015), such as children in care and care leavers (Stein, 2006). This should also be seen in light of Bowlby's attachment theory (1988, 1998), highlighting the importance of a secure and trusting mother–infant bond on the development and mental health of the child (see also Ainsworth et al., 2015). Houston (2010) argues in favour of a critical realist perspective in child welfare research, treating Bowlby's theory of attachment and maternal deprivation as primary evidence of the fact that emotions are pre-discursive (see also Trillingsgaard et al., 2011).

However, what is 'real' (and 'non-discursive') here is always debatable. Drawing on the social constructionist viewpoint, it could be argued that Bowlby's theory has been produced (and interpreted) from a traditional viewpoint, supporting the fact that caring for the family is a mother's fundamental duty. As such, his theory is not necessarily evidence of the fact that emotions are pre-discursive. Instead, it can be understood as an example of how psychology is a powerful institution that is responsible for creating and maintaining dominant constructions of child development in society.

Historiography on the institutional and intellectual context of Bowlby's ideas has ranged widely in focus. Polat (2016), for example, highlights how some focus upon the social and economic factors that contributed to the intellectual climate in which attachment theory acquired traction, whilst others looked at the intellectual affinities and differences between Bowlby's theory and the prevailing views in post-WWI British psychiatry. A critical realist perspective, and the ontological premise therein – that the world exists and is real, but that investigations of it are saturated with interests and values – thus offers a route through which to engage with and evaluate both perspectives of Bowlby's theory. This ties in with what Bhaskar (2014) refers to as 'holistic causality', i.e. the fact that what happens to one element, and between members of a complex, affects the other.

Bhaskar and Danermark (2006) and Collier (2003) use the term 'laminated systems' to mark the irreducibility of mechanisms at different levels, for example in relation to the World Health Organization's (WHO) notion of a human being as, for health purposes, a bio-psycho-social mix. Yet, although the holistic perspective put forward by the biopsychosocial model (Engel, 1980) can be seen as complementary to a CR approach to safeguarding and mental health and wellbeing, it also falls short of engaging with a central aspiration of critical realism. This refers to the integration and balance of ontological realism, epistemological relativism and judgemental rationality (Patel & Pilgrim, 2018; Pilgrim, 2015). For example, whilst the biopsychosocial model sheds light on the interaction of biomedical, sociological and psychological factors in relation to mental health problems such as depression, it treats the diagnostic criteria and related concepts, e.g. 'schizophrenia' and 'depression', as accurate medical facts (Pilgrim, 2015). Yet mental health illness, safeguarding and child protection are tied to – and a product of – contexts (and related interpretations) of inequality and complexity, such as trauma and loss, as well as political factors across time and space.

From this vantage point it could be argued that diagnosis of mental health issues, related criteria and language needs to be critically evaluated and scrutinised as well. By overlooking this, the biopsychosocial model could be perceived as simply reinforcing biological reductionism, albeit through a more applied or adjusted lens (Pilgrim, 2015). Critical realism and its focus on retroductive reasoning, on the other hand, allows for a critique of the way in which child abuse, neglect and mental health issues are conceptualised, and instead turns to the conditions under which variations in behaviour and the expression of distress are described in one way rather than another.

As well as taking account of embodied conditions (such as trauma or stress) and material conditions (such as individual means and resources to access services), approaches regarding child protection, safeguarding and mental health support in childhood also need to be seen in light of wider institutional factors, including the post-industrial, neoliberal austerity context in which cuts have effected long-term established services. For example, the available budget for local authority children's centres and services has fallen by more than a third since the start of the 2010s (Morton, 2013).

Children's centres are a UK government initiative introduced in 1998 to provide a range of services for parents and young children in deprived areas (with a focus on health, mental health, family support and employment). Research shows that children's centres play a role in improving the mental health of mothers and the functioning of families, yet benefits are being eroded by cuts (Torjesen, 2016). In addition to this there is evidence that Child and Adolescent Mental Health Services (CAMHS) budgets have been cut as well since 2010, and spending on adult care is also affected (Taylor-Gooby & Stoker, 2011).

Generally, public spending on children's services is low. For example, there is evidence that Government spending on children at risk of abuse and neglect has been slashed by more than a quarter since 2015. According to Turner et al. (2015) a historical narrative structured around rights (the right to health and the right to liberty), instigated by the introduction of the NHS in 1948 and the establishment of the welfare state, is now complicated by the rise of new organising categories such as 'costs', 'risks', 'needs', 'inclusion' and 'equality' – leading to competing visions regarding child protection, safeguarding provision and mental health support. It follows that discursive, material and embodied factors are important and can be treated as both autonomous and interconnected (e.g. austerity is an institutional discourse that has material effects).

Moreover, this is where critical realism can assist in shedding light on conditions and causal factors associated with the workings of the deserving/undeserving paradigm. I argue that, at a time of ever-increasing thresholds for access and cuts to resources, one can see a contemporary manifestation of the punitive deserving/undeserving paradigm, inherited from the 1834 New Poor Law and the 19th-century child rescue movement in order to justify who is 'entitled' to help and who is not. Here, 'worthiness', 'deservedness' and perceived entitlement to support are all too often linked to behaviour and lifestyle choices, suggesting that some children – due to unmanageable behaviour and bad lifestyle choices (such as in the sexual exploitation scandals discussed in Chapter 1) – are beyond help. Yet, this suggests that some children may be 'good', 'bad', 'moral' or 'immoral' by choice, and negates the fact that early trauma, neglect and mental health issues in childhood can all play a role here. For example, there is evidence of a correlation between childhood mistreatment and anti-social behaviour, representing a complex interaction between genes and environment (Ellis, 2020; Leckman et al., 2007).

This confusion around terms is not something new. For example, notions of morality and the ability to distinguish between choosing good and evil, and related behaviour, were concerns of psychiatrists and physicians (such as Rush, Prichard, Kraepelin and Maudsley) in the 19th and early 20th centuries, and confusion caused by unclear terms persists today. As discussed in Chapter 1, an example of this is the ambiguous portrayal of 'callous and unemotional' children in the media, as if this is a given and some children are just 'born bad'. I argue that, by exploring past and present voices of young people and practitioners simultaneously, it is possible to provide insight into per-ceptions, constructs, structures and mechanisms that have been shaped by long-term and immediate factors (e.g. institutional, political and material). Here I am specifically interested in manifestations of the deserving/undeserving paradigm in the late 1800s and the 21st century (as both periods are marked by a purge on public spending) and how this is understood by young people and safeguarding professionals. Below I will explore this further by providing insights into how I applied and embedded critical realism into my specific research, drawing on historic and contemporary datasets.

2.4 Applying critical realism to historical and contemporary datasets

Despite significant research on safeguarding and mental health in childhood, either with a focus on historic or present data, there is no research that literally places current and past datasets next to each other, comparing and contrasting conditions and structures simulta-neously. Yet, such a focus is important in making sense of current and past practices, also in light of the legacy of the deserving/undeserving paradigm in child safeguarding and mental health support decisions. In an attempt to provide services where there are ever-increasing thresh-olds for access and cuts to resources, the deserving/undeserving para-digm reflects a historic and contemporary justification for who is 'entitled' to help and who is not. Self–Other distinctions are central to social and temporal spaces and identities, and research shows that specific social groups – e.g. children in care, young care leavers, people with mental illness – are often presented as the 'Other' (Knaak et al., 2017; Roberts & Schiavenato, 2017; Sims-Schouten et al., 2019).

Child protection is fundamentally political because of the broad range of definitions associated with this; representing this as happening to 'others' rather than oneself is one way in which this is portrayed. Chauhan and Foster (2014) argue that 'Othering' is achieved through three distinct representational pathways: representational absence, representations of difference and representations of threat. I aim to provide insights into the quandary between the three: 'absence' (under-representation and under-privilege, highlighting a possible need for a critical focus); 'difference' (stigma and labels); and 'threat' (e.g. financial, moral) – instigating both a 'caring philanthropic approach' and judgements in relation to 'deservedness'.

The tenets of critical realism encourage a focus on the interaction between structure and agency in stratified entities, viewing context or situational influences as crucial to an understanding of processes and emergent outcomes (Kessler & Bach, 2014; Saka-Helmhout, 2014). This is different to the focus on generalisable laws postulated by positivists, or the emphasis on lived experiences or beliefs of social actors inherent in interpretivism. My goal is to provide insight into practices and perceptions regarding the most vulnerable children, referred to by Stein (2006) as 'victims' – a term for the most disadvantaged children who have spent time in care, have complex needs and have had damaging pre-care family experiences. Critical realism provides insight into oppression, inequality and uneven practices through the search for generative mechanisms and causal factors, which combined might have created a phenomenon over time, and within this influences particular outcomes and practices (Mutch, 2014; Sims-Schouten et al., 2019). For example, historically, biomedical theories centralising notions of inheritance and biological determinism in relation to 'mental deficiency' may have encouraged the belief that some individuals were biologically disadvantaged, degenerate and beyond help (Pilgrim, 2014).

As can be seen from Chapter 1, 'idiot, 'idiocy' and 'imbecility' were common diagnoses for those under the age of ten in the 19th century (Sohasky, 2015). Moreover, links were made between heredity, moral development and psychopathology in childhood (Hall, 1904); and there is evidence that 'moral competence' and 'moral incompetence' are terms that are still applied to child behaviour today (Sims-Schouten et al., 2019). Thus there is a need to gain insight into the quandary between the three structural concepts outlined above: 'absence' (under-representation/under-privilege and what is missing in a context or institution/organisation, highlighting a possible need for a critical focus); 'difference' (stigma/labels in relation to 'bad behaviour' and mental illness); and 'threat' (e.g. high cost of services, 'immoral behaviour').

This book draws on a historic and contemporary dataset that will be analysed in light of the critical realist ontology discussed above. The first consists of archival data, namely 108 case files from the Waifs and Strays Society (now the Children's Society) representing the correspondence and perceptions of custodians, doctors and other professionals, as well as children and parents between 1881 and 1918. Over 20,000 children were looked after by the Waifs and Strays Society between its creation in 1881 and the end of the First World War. Case files were selected through keywords with a specific focus on mental health, wellbeing, abuse, neglect and behaviour. The second dataset comprises of contemporary data, and consists of semi-structured interviews with 24 young care leavers and 22 safeguarding practitioners/professionals; the interviews focused on safeguarding and mental health and the wellbeing of care leavers. Drawing on critical realist ontology, I compared and contrasted the datasets in order to gain insight into historically conditioned perceptions and practices in relation to safeguarding and mental health in childhood. Here, I was specifically interested in generative (non-linear) mechanisms regarding long-term factors (such as institutional, psychological and political) and shorter-term factors (e.g. demographics and geographical location).

Drawing on my previous work with a focus on applied critical realism, the current research is grounded in three broad phases (see also Sims-Schouten et al., 2007, 2019; Sims-Schouten & Riley, 2014, 2018). The first phase consists of an in-depth analysis of primary, secondary and grey literature, as well as policy documents, to identify entities that may combine to form causal factors and generative mechanisms that (could) play a role in mental health support and safeguarding in childhood, now and in late Victorian times. I call this the 'discovery' phase, but this can also be referred to (in terms of critical realist language) as 'retroduction', as discussed earlier in this chapter. Phase 1 focuses on developing the broadest possible understanding of what factors (individual, embodied, material and institutional) might be relevant to the experiences and sense making of the participants in the datasets, as well as testing this iteratively against new information (see also Cromby & Nightingale, 1999).

The focus on discovery and retroduction of phase 1 is different to a regular literature review, which provides the theoretical basis for a piece of research and determines the nature of the research. Instead, phase one focuses on identifying the most common reoccurring elements that may impact on the participants in the datasets (e.g. psychological and political as well as contextual structures) (see also Sims-Schouten & Riley, 2018). In addition to providing insight into possible (non-linear) generative mechanisms and causal factors in relation to child safeguarding practices and mental health support, phase one also informs the analysis and keywords of the historic and contemporary datasets (i.e. the archival research and topics for the semi-structured interviews.

The next phase is the data analysis phase, which involves thematic content analysis of the historic and contemporary data in order to identify themes within each dataset and compare patterns and contrasts within and across the sets (Sims-Schouten et al., 2019). Thematic content analysis is useful when it comes to gaining insight into the thematic content of both interview transcripts and texts by identifying common themes (Anderson, 2004). Specifically, thematic content analysis allows for both a quantification of data (drawing on content analysis and its focus on measuring the frequency of different categories) and a qualifying narrative focus (through thematic analysis) (Vaismoradi et al., 2013). Drawing on thematic content analysis, I identified a common list of themes, and grouped and distilled this from the data in order to provide insight into the communality of voices across the participants; this will be discussed further in Chapters 3 and 4.

The final stage, phase 3, specifically focuses on applying the critical realist aspect, namely by examining the data in terms of how participants' personal/individual, material and institutional contexts (informed by phase 1) may provide the conditions for sense-making. For example, what may be relevant to both datasets described are early experiences of insecure attachment, child abuse and the close association between lack of support networks, low socio-economic status and mental health problems (Boath et al., 2013; Robb et al., 2013). This shows how elements of embodiment, materiality and institutions overlap and interact.

Both datasets are analysed alongside each other, using vertical (going through each extract, file, interview on its own 'vertically') and horizontal (comparing key concepts and emerging themes in the datasets by literally putting them next to each other) as analysis strategies. The following themes (running across both datasets) are the result of the in-depth analysis described above: 'beyond help'; 'child/family needs as central'; 'problematic children, mental health issues'; 'problematic children, behavioural issues'; 'child abuse and neglect'; 'sexual abuse and sexualised behaviour'; 'grateful'; 'I used to be bad'. These will be explored further in Chapters 3 and 4.

Conclusion

In this chapter I have provided a case for using and applying critical realist ontology in order to make sense of practices and perceptions with a focus on mental health support and safeguarding in childhood. This applied critical realist approach draws on my previous work (Sims-Schouten et al., 2007; Sims-Schouten & Riley, 2014, 2018), as well as the work of Bhaskar (1989, 2014) and Pilgrim (2014, 2015). I have shown how critical realism, as a metatheory, uses elements from both social constructionism and biomedical realism. As such, critical realism can form the basis for research with a focus on making sense of child protection practices, taking account of the fact that these practices and related perceptions with regard to safeguarding and mental illness are both socially constructed as well as influenced by external factors and forces that can be real and independent of any one person or social group (Sayer, 2000). My research starts from the premise that the principles of 'less or more eligibility' lie at the heart of the British welfare system, both now and in historic times. These principles appear to affect the children and families with the most complex mental health and safeguarding needs the most.

Stein (2006, 277) has suggested that there are three broad groups of care leavers, characterised as those who are 'moving on', 'survivors' and 'victims'. The 'moving on' group are likely to have had some stability and continuity in their lives, including positive experiences whilst in care and some educational success before leaving care. The group referred to as 'survivors' are not as fortunate as the 'moving on' group in that they are likely to have experienced more instability and disruption whilst in care, and gained few educational qualifications. 'Victims' are the most disadvantaged group, with the most damaging pre-care family experiences, disruption and instability whilst in care and post-care, and complex mental health needs and problems. It is the latter group ('victims') that this research focuses on. The next two chapters, respectively, will provide an overview of their experiences in late Victorian times and contemporary times.

References

Ainsworth, M.D.S., Blehar, M.C., Waters, E. and Wall, S.N. (2015). *Patterns of Attachment: A Psychological Study of the Strange Situation*. Hove: Psychology Press.

Anderson, R. (2004). Intuitive inquiry: an epistemology of the heart for scientific inquiry. *Humanistic Psychologist*, 32(4), 307–341.

Bhaskar, R. (1989). *Reclaiming Reality*. London: Verso.

Bhaskar, R. (2014). Foreword. In: Edwards, P., O.Mahoney, J. and Vincent, S. (Eds.), *Studying Organizations Using Critical Realism: A Practical Guide.* Oxford: Oxford University Press, v–xv.

Bhaskar, R. and Danermark, B. (2006). Metatheory, interdisciplinarity and disability research: a critical realist perspective. *Scandinavian Journal of Disability Research*, 8(4), 278–297, doi:10.1080/15017410600914329.

Boath, E.H., Henshaw, C. and Bradley, E. (2013). Meeting the challenges of teenage mothers with postpartum depression: overcoming stigma through support. *Journal of Reproductive and Infant Psychology*, 31(4), 352–369. doi:10.1080/02646838.2013.800635.

Bowlby, J. (1988). *A Secure Base: Parent-Child Attachment and Healthy Human Development.* London: Routledge.

Bowlby, J. (1998). *Attachment and Loss* (Vol. 3). London: Random House.

Brady, G., Lowe, P. and Lauritzen, S.O. (Eds.) (2015). *Children, Health and Well-Being: Policy Debates and Lived Experience.* Hoboken, NJ: Wiley.

Carrillo, A. (2018). Using structural social work theory to drive anti-oppressive practice with Latino immigrants. *Advances in Social Work*, 18(3). doi:10.18060/21663.

Chauhan, A. and Foster, J. (2014). Representations of poverty in British newspapers: a case of 'othering' the threat? *Journal of Community and Applied Social Psychology*, 24(5), 390–405.

Collier, A. (2003). Dialectic in Marxism and critical realism. In: Brown, A., Fleetwood, S. and Roberts, J.M. (Eds.), *Critical Realism and Marxism.* London: Routledge, 155–168.

Cooklin, A.R., Giallo, R. and Rose, N. (2012). Parental fatigue and parenting practices during early childhood: an Australian community survey. *Child: Care, Health and Development*, 38(5), 654–664. doi:10.1111/j.1365-2214. 2011.01333.x.

Cradock, G. (2014). Who owns child abuse? *Social Sciences*, 3, 854–870.

Cromby, J. (2016). Developing schizophrenia. *Theory & Psychology*, 26(5), 607–619.

Cromby, J. and Harper, D.J. (2009). Paranoia: a social account. *Theory & Psychology*, 19(3), 335–361. doi:10.1177/0959354309104158.

Cromby, J., and Nightingale, D.J. (1999). What's wrong with social constructionism? In Nightingale, D.J. and Cromby, J. (Eds.), *Social Constructionist Psychology: A Critical Analysis of Theory and Practice.* Buckingham: Open University Press, 1–19.

Deacon, B.J. (2013). The biomedical model of mental disorder: a critical analysis of its validity, utility, and effects on psychotherapy research. *Clinical Psychology Review*, 33(7), 846–861.

Dunning, M.J. and Giallo, R. (2012). Fatigue, parenting stress, self-efficacy and satisfaction in mothers of infants and young children. *Journal of Reproductive and Infant Psychology*, 30(2), 145–159. doi:10.1080/02646838.2012.693910.

Ellis, K. (2020). Blame and culpability in children's narratives of sexual abuse. *Child Abuse Review*, 28(6), 405–417.

Engel, G.L. (1980). The clinical application of the biopsychosocial model. *American Journal of Psychiatry*, 137(5), 535–544. doi:10.1176/ajp.137.5.535.

Fitzpatrick, S. (2005). Explaining homelessness: a critical realist perspective. *Housing, Theory and Society*, 22(1), 1–17.

Gergen, K.J. (2009). *Relational Being: Beyond Self and Community*. New York: Oxford University Press.

Gingell, K. (2001). The forgotten children: children admitted to a county asylum between 1854 and 1900, *Psychiatric Bulletin*, 25, 432–434.

Hacking, I. (1991), The making and molding of child abuse. *Critical Inquiry*, 17(2), 253–288.

Hall, G. Stanley (1904). *Adolescence: Its Psychology and Its relations to Physiology, Anthropology, Sociology, Sex, Crime, Religion and Education*. New York: Appleton,

Houston, S. (2010). Prising open the black box: critical realism, action research and social work. *Qualitative Social Work*, 9(1), 73–91. doi:10.1177/1473325009355622.

Kessler, I. and Bach, S. (2014). Comparing cases. In: Edwards, P.K., O'Mahoney, J. and Vincent, S. (Eds.), *Studying Organizations Using Critical Realism: A Practical Guide*. Oxford: Oxford University Press, 168–184.

Klin, A. and Jones, W. (2007). Embodied psychoanalysis? Or, on the influence of psychodynamic theory and developmental science. In: Mayes, L., Fonagy, P. and Target, M. (Eds.), *Developmental Science and Psychanalysis*. London: Karnac, 5–38.

Knaak, S., Mantler, E. and Szeto, A. (2017). Mental illness-related stigma in healthcare. *Healthcare Management Forum*, 32(2), 111–116.

Leckman, J.F., Feldman, R. and Swain, J.E. (2007). Primary parental preoccupation: revisited. In: Mayes, L., Fonagy, P. and Target, M. (Eds.), *Developmental Science and Psychanalysis*. London: Karnac, 89–108.

Lysaker, P.H., Gumley, A., Brüne, M., Vanheule, S., Buck, K.D. and Dimaggio, G. (2011). Deficits in the ability to recognize one's own affects and those of others: associations with neurocognition, symptoms and sexual trauma among persons with schizophrenia spectrum disorders. *Consciousness and Cognition*, 20, 1183–1192.

Mahoney, M.J. and Granvold, D.K. (2005). Constructivism and psychotherapy. *World Psychiatry*, 4(2), 74–77.

McNamee, S. and Gergen, K.J. (Eds.) (1992). *Therapy as Social Construction*. London: Sage.

Melling, J., Adair, R. and Forsythe, B. (1997). 'A proper lunatic for two years': pauper lunatic children in Victorian and Edwardian England. Child admissions to the Devon County Asylum, 1845–1914. *Journal of Social History*, 31(2), 371–394.

Morrison, J. (2016). *Familiar Strangers, Juvenile Panics and the British Press: The Decline of Social Trust*. London: Palgrave Macmillan.

Morton, S. (2014). *Wisdom, Justice, Charity. Canadian Social Welfare through the Life of Jane B. Wisdom 1884–1975*. Toronto: University of Toronto Press.

Mullaly, R.P. (1993). *Structural Social Work: Ideology, Theory and Practice.* Toronto: McClelland & Stewart.

Mutch, A. (2014). History and documents in critical realism. In: Edwards, P., O'Mahoney, J. and Vincent, S. (Eds.), *Studying Organizations Using Critical Realism: A Practical Guide.* Oxford: Oxford University Press, 223–240.

O'Mahoney, J. and Vincent, S. (2014). Critical realism as an empirical project: a beginner's guide. In: Edwards, P., O'Mahoney, J. and Vincent, S. (Eds.), *Studying Organizations Using Critical Realism: A Practical Guide.* Oxford: Oxford University Press, 1–20.

Patel, N. and Pilgrim, D. (2018). Psychologists and torture: critical realism as a resource for analysis and training. *Journal of Critical Realism,* 7(2), 176–191.

Payne. M. (2011). *Humanistic Social Work (Core Principles in Practice).* Chicago: Lyceum.

Pilgrim, D. (2014). Some implications of critical realism for mental health research. *Social Theory & Health,* 12(1), 1–12.

Pilgrim, D. (2015). The biopsychosocial model in health research: its strengths and limitations for critical realists. *Journal of Critical Realism,* 14(2), 164–180.

Pilgrim, D. and Bentall, R. (1999). The medicalisation of misery: a critical realist analysis of the concept of depression. *Journal of Mental Health,* 8(3), 261–274. doi:10.1080/09638239917427.

Polat, B. (2016). Before attachment theory: separation research at the Tavistock Clinic, 1948–1956. *Journal of the History of Behavioral Sciences,* 53(1), 48–70.

Robb, Y., McIncry, D. and Hollins Martin, C.J. (2013). Exploration of the experiences of young mothers seeking and accessing health services. *Journal of Reproductive and Infant Psychology,* 31(4), 399–412. doi:10.1080/02646838.2013.832181.

Roberts, J.M. (2014). Critical realism, dialectics, and qualitative research methods. *Journal of the Theory of Social Behaviour,* 44(1), 1–23. doi:10.1111/jtsb.12056.

Roberts, M.L.M. and Schiavenato, M. (2017). Othering in the nursing context: a concept analysis. *Nursing Open,* 4, 174–181.

Saka-Helmhout, A. (2014). Critical realism and international comparative case research. In: Edwards, P.K., O'Mahoney, J. and Vincent, S. (Eds.), *Studying Organizations Using Critical Realism: A Practical Guide.* Oxford: Oxford University Press, 185–204.

Sayer A. (2000) *Realism and Social Science.* London: Sage.

Scambler, G. and Scambler, S. (2015). Theorizing health inequalities: the untapped potential of dialectical critical realism. *Social Theory & Health,* 13, 340–354.

Schalinski, I., Fischer, Y., and Rockstroh, B. (2015). Impact of childhood adversities on the short-term course of illness in psychotic spectrum disorders. *Psychiatry Research,* 228(3), 633–640.

Sims-Schouten, W. and Hayden, C., (2017). Mental health and wellbeing of care leavers: making sense of their perspectives. *Child & Family Social Work*, 24(4), 1480–1487.

Sims-Schouten, W. and Riley, S. (2018). Presenting critical realist discourse analysis as a tool for making sense of service users' accounts of their mental health problems. *Qualitative Health Research*, 29(7). doi:10.1177/1049732318818824.

Sims-Schouten, W. and Riley, S.E. (2014). Employing a form of critical realist discourse analysis for identity research: an example from women's talk of motherhood, childcare and employment. In: Edwards, P., O'Mahoney, J. and Vincent, S. (Eds.), *Studying Organizations Using Critical Realism: A Practical Guide*. Oxford: Oxford University Press, 46–65.

Sims-Schouten, W., Riley, S.C.E. and Willig, C. (2007). Critical realism: a presentation of a systematic method of analysis using women's talk of motherhood, childcare and female employment as an example. *Theory & Psychology*, 17(1), 127–150.

Sims-Schouten, W., Skinner, A. and Rivett, K. (2019). Child safeguarding in light of the deserving/undeserving paradigm: a historical and contemporary analysis. *Child Abuse & Neglect*, 94. doi:10.1016/j.chiabu.2019.104025.

Sohasky, K.E. (2015). Safeguarding the interests of the state from defective delinquent girls. *Journal of the History of Behavioral Sciences*, 52(1), 20–40. doi:10.1002/jhbs.21765.

Stein, M. (2006). Research review: young people leaving care. *Child and Family Social Work*, 11(3), 273–279.

Taylor, S.J. (2016). *Child Insanity in England, 1845–1907*. Basingstoke: Palgrave Macmillan.

Taylor-Gooby, P. and Stoker, G. (2011). The Coalition Programme: a new vision for Britain or politics as usual? *Political Quarterly*, 82(1), 4–15. doi:10.1111/j.1467-1923X.2011.02169.x/full.

Torjesen, I. (2016). Austerity cuts are eroding benefit of Sure Start children's centres, *BMJ*, 352, i335. doi:10.1136/bmj.i335.

Trillingsgaard, T., Elklit, A., Shevlin, M. and Maimburg, R.D. (2011). Adult attachment at the transition to motherhood: predicting worry, health care utility and relationship functioning. *Journal of Reproductive and Infant Psychology*, 29(4), 354–363. doi:10.1080/02646838.2011.611937.

Turner, J., Hayward, R., Angel, K., Fulford, B., Hall, J., Millard, C. and Thomson, M. (2015). The History of mental health services in modern England: practitioner memories and the direction of future research. *Medical History*, 59(4), 599–624. doi:10.1017/mdh.2015.48.

Vaismoradi, M., Turunen, H. and Bondas, T. (2013). Content analysis and thematic analysis: implications for conducting a qualitative descriptive study. *Nursing & Health Sciences*, 15, 398–405.

White, M. (2011). *Narrative Practice: Continuing the Conversations*. New York: Norton.

Wilson, N. (2020). *The Space that Separates: A Realist Theory of Art*. Abingdon: Routledge.

3 The case of the Waifs and Strays Society (1881–1918)

During the latter decades of the 19th century child support, protection and safeguarding were organised through a combination of state services and voluntary agencies. One such voluntary or philanthropic agency was the Waifs and Strays Society, established in 1881 by Edward Rudolf (Higginbotham, 2017; Skinner & Thomas, 2018). The central goal of the Waifs and Strays Society was to set up homes for destitute children in connection with the Church of England that, as far as possible, would provide children with a family environment rather than an institutional one (Higginbotham, 2017). Now known as the Children's Society, the agency has become one of Britain's leading child support agencies.

In this chapter, I will shed light on the practices and language around safeguarding and mental health in case files of children supported and taken into care by the Waifs and Strays Society during the first 37 years of its existence, from its inception in 1881 until 1918 (in line with the 100-year Data Protection Act). Over 20,000 children from across England and Wales were cared for by the Waifs and Strays Society between 1881 and the end of the First World War. The children's case files consist of correspondence highlighting the perception of custodians, educators, medical officers, church officials, practitioners linked to asylums and industrial schools, parents and children (during and after care). Drawing on critical realist ontology and thematic content analysis, introduced in Chapter 2, this chapter will critically analyse causal mechanisms that generate events (in a non-linear and stratified way), how these events are experienced by individuals, and processes and support mechanisms in place or missing (Bhaskar, 2014; Sims-Schouten et al., 2019; Vaismoradi et al., 2013).

3.1 Children's case files: 'mental health', 'behaviour', 'abuse' and 'wretched families'

As discussed in Chapters 1 and 2, I am specifically interested in the group of children classified as 'victims' (Stein, 2006) – young people with complex (mental health) needs and damaging care experiences (pre- as well as post-care). Moreover, I am also interested in how the needs of and support for those children are discussed and addressed in the correspondence linked to the case files. This includes language around 'deservedness/undeservedness', and that some children are 'unfit', 'unmanageable', 'unsatisfactory' and 'unsuitable'; it also includes examples of correspondence and language around the child's mental wellbeing and behaviour and related support mechanisms. I selected relevant children's case files through searches of the Children's Society online database 'Hidden Lives Revealed' and archive catalogue using specific keywords, such as 'mental' and 'behaviour', which will be discussed in more detail below.[1] A total of 108 children's case files were selected: 69 were girls and 39 were boys; their average age was 10 years old at the time of the application to the Waifs and Strays Society, with the youngest 2 years old and the oldest 16. Reasons given for being taken on by the Waifs and Strays Society included: the fact that both parents were dead (in 12 of the case files); the mother had died and the father was unable to care for the child (17 cases); the father had died (33 cases); or one parent was in a mental asylum (in 22 of the cases, 14 of which mentioned the mother in this context). The remainder of the applications to the Waifs and Strays referred to 'wretched families' and 'dysfunctional homes' as reasons the child had been taken into care, as shown in see Table 3.1. The case files were examined during visits to the Children's Society archives in London.

The search for keywords was informed by historic writings, historiography and history literature/research (see Chapters 1 and 2). For example, common diagnoses for those under the age of ten include 'idiocy' and 'imbecility', but did not necessarily indicate cognitive deficiencies. Instead, 'idiocy' was seen as an example of reversion to a lower level in the evolutionary scale. At the same time, as was discussed in Chapter 1, from the end of the 19th century it became more widely acknowledged that juvenile insanity and 'madness' in children was different from 'mental retardation' and epilepsy (Sampson, 1976; Rey et al., 2015; Stewart, 2011). The search for keywords in relation to 'mental', 'mental health' and 'mental deficiency' resulted in 60 hits (44 girls, 16 boys), relating to the following terms: mental illness; depressed; lunatic; insane anxiety; mental deficiency; mental condition;

Table 3.1 Children's case files information

Total number of cases	108
Gender	69 girls, 39 boys
Age at application	2–16 years
Reason for acceptance by Waifs and Strays	Both parents died: N=12 Mother died: N=17 Father died: N=33 Mother in mental asylum: N=14 Father in mental asylum: N=8 'Dysfunctional' or 'wretched' home: N=30
Admittance to mental asylum	Under the age of 18: N=13 (10 girls; 3 boys) From age 18: N=7 (6 girls; 1 boy) Both from below 18 and after turning 18: N=5 (all girls)
Cases with correspondence from young person included	N=18 (aged 10–50)
Cases with correspondence regarding post-care provision	N=34 (asylums; homes; employers; after-care association; Girls Welfare Department)

mental capacity; mental trouble; unsound mind; acute mania; hysterical; melancholia; nervous breakdown; neurotic condition; imbecile; sensitivities; delicate nature.

I was also interested in the language around behavioural issues, as literature and research indicates that behavioural disorders were largely considered moral issues and problems, and the result of 'badness' rather than 'madness', and deserving of punishment (e.g. Sohasky, 2015; see also Chapter 1). I used the following keywords here: 'bad' behaviour, 'temper', 'unmanageable' – which resulted in 45 hits (26 girls and 19 boys). In 18 of the cases (15 girls and 3 boys) both mental health issues and bad behaviour were addressed in the files. Child abuse and neglect including sexual abuse were mentioned in 27 of the case files (18 girls, 9 boys). Sexual abuse and 'sexualised behaviour' was only discussed in relation to girls (13 cases). In a total of 25 cases reference was made to admittance to a mental asylum: 13 children (10 females and 3 males) spent time in a asylum before they turned 18 years old; 7 (1 male and 6 females) spent time in an asylum from age 18 onwards; and with 5 children (all female) there was both talk of entering an asylum prior to and after they were 18 years old.

A total of 18 files (for 11 females and 7 males) contained correspondence from the young people whilst they were in care and post-care (spanning the ages 10–50 years). Moreover, in 34 of the case files correspondence regarding post-care provision/employment (where all the young people involved had reached the age of 18) was included, from asylums, homes, employers, after-care associations and the Girls Welfare Department.

In line with the critical realist approach, the next section sheds light on the non-linear causal structures and mechanisms in relation to institutional factors, social policy and psychology/psychiatry of the time.

3.2 Institutional/organisational factors, social policy/social work and psychology/psychiatry of the time

As discussed in Chapter 2, the present research draws on critical realism and is grounded in three phases (see also Sims-Schouten et al., 2019). Phase 1 turns to published research, policy documents and 'grey' literature with the aim of identifying some of the entities that may combine to form causal factors, in this case in relation to the constructs and realities of safeguarding and mental health and mental illness in childhood. In line with phase 1 and the critical realist ontology discussed in Chapter 2, an in-depth and focused review of relevant (historic and contemporary) literature, policy documents and secondary data was undertaken to identify the most common elements of embodiment, institutions and materiality impacting the participants. Table 3.2 summarises the outcome of phase 1 of the study and provides examples of psychological and political structures and institutions, as well as contextual factors in relation to the current dataset (but note that this table is by no means exhaustive). In line with the critical realist approach discussed earlier, these factors reflect non-linear dynamics and generative mechanisms that may or may not be activated, depending on conditions.

Phase 2 of the research comprises thematic content analysis of the 108 children's case files in order to identify themes and patters and contrasts across the datasets. A number of key themes were identified across both datasets, and details relating to the historic dataset are summarised in Table 3.3.

Finally, phase 3 introduces the critical realist aspect by examining the data in light of personal, material and institutional contexts (informed by phase 1). Below, drawing on this three-phase critical realist analysis, I will discuss and analyse examples of case files in light of the themes outlined in Table 3.3. Note that I have used pseudonyms (some case files lack names), although all files are available through the Children's Society online databases.[2]

Table 3.2 Institutions/organisations, social policy/social work and psychology/psychiatry factors: dataset 1 – Waifs and Strays Society/Children's Society (1881–1918)

Institution/organisation	Social policy/social work	Psychology/psychiatry
New Poor Law (1834) workhouse Industrial schools (caring for neglected children), 1857–1933; Barnardo's, charity for the care of vulnerable children, founded by Thomas John Barnardo in 1866 Waifs & Strays Society, child care agency, established by Edward Rudolf in 1881 Asylums (no age limit); no specialist children's services with regard to mental health support	Charity Organisation Society (1869): system of personal social work; instigated by George Goschen (president of the Poor Law Board) following the slashing of Poor Law spending in 1869 NSPCC established in 1884 The Prevention of Cruelty to and Protection of Children Act, or 'Children's Charter', established in 1889	Emphasis on heredity (e.g. Maudsley, 1879) Growing understanding of multiple factors involved in childhood wellbeing, and the development of childhood psychiatric disorders

Sources: Action for Children et al., 2017; Bazalgette et al., 2015; Gingell, 2001; Hacking, 1991; Higginbotham, 2017; Maudsley, 1879; Melling et al., 1997; Rey et al., 2015; Sims-Schouten et al., 2019; Ward, 1990.

Table 3.3 Key themes in correspondence about and by the child

Theme	Correspondence about the child (N=108)	Correspondence by the child (N=18: 11 girls, 7 boys)
'Beyond help' (unmanageable, unsuitable, unsatisfactory, uncontrollable, unfit)	46% (N=50)	–
Centralising the needs of the child	19% (N=20)	–
Mental health issues (a problematic child)	56% (N=60: 44 girls; 16 boys)	11% (N=2 girls)
Behavioural issues (a problematic child)	42% (N=45: 26 girls, 19 boys)	5% (N=1 boy)

(*continued*)

Table 3.3 (continued)

Theme	Correspondence about the child (N=108)	Correspondence by the child (N=18: 11 girls, 7 boys)
Mental health & behaviour issues both mentioned	17% (N=18: 15 girls, 3 boys)	–
Child abuse & neglect	25% (N=27: 18 girls, 9 boys)	5% (N=1 girl)
Sexual abuse/sexualised behaviour	12% (N=13, all girls)	–
'Grateful'	–	44% (N=8: 5 girls, 3 boys)
I am/used to be 'bad'	–	33% (N=6: 5 girls, 1 boy)

3.3 Maud (case file 1269): beyond help, unfit, behavioural issues and of a low moral type

Maud was born in 1874 and the application to the Waifs and Strays Society was made in 1888, when she was 14 years old. Not much is known about her early life, although the application notes that Maud herself divulged that her father had once been a soldier in the 77th Regiment in India. Later her father was an itinerant china mender and beggar. Her mother died when Maud was about 3½, and following this she was placed in Barnsley workhouse; her father removed her from the workhouse in 1879, on his second marriage. There is talk about Maud's father and stepmother abusing and starving her, and that following this Maud ran away and ended up in Wakefield Preventative House in March 1887. This was not a Waifs and Strays home, yet correspondence between Wakefield and the Society is included in the file, suggesting that Maud was considered untruthful and a bad influence on other girls. In the application to the Waifs and Strays that follows in 1888, there is some acknowledgement of Maud's unfortunate background and pre-care experiences – 'X's father and stepmother abused and starved her', as well as:

> I wrote to an address of a friend of the girl in Sheffield who had shown the girl kindness & she corroborated the girl had said of her life there & said she was very badly treated & starved by her father & stepmother. Since they began itinerating she had known nothing of them.

Yet, Maud is also described as 'behaving badly' and being 'of a low moral type herself', and that she uses 'bad language':

> [Maud] says they were always moving from town to town walking long distances, & taking lodgings as cheap as they could, begging their food during the day. There is no doubt she is accustomed to life in low lodging houses, & is of a low moral type herself, using bad language & acquainted with evil in many ways. She had run away from her father in Leeds when she came to us & brought in with her, a large quantity of bread & scraps which she had begged on the way.

The application continues: 'She reads & sews nicely & is affectionate, but is very deceitful & untruthful & utterly unfit from a moral point of view to have charge of children.'

Following her application to the Waifs and Strays in 1888, Maud is sent to the Fareham Home for Girls (Hampshire) in April 1888. In June 1890 she is then sent out to work with a family in Sydenham, London, but steals from them and behaves badly; consequently, she is sent back to Fareham in October of the same year. Maud is sent into service in two other places, but they also return her to Fareham because of bad behaviour. This, together with the fact that she is a runaway and 'acquainted with evil in many ways', means that she is seen as beyond help and unfit. This is reiterated by various employers; for example Maud's first employer writes the following in a letter to the Waifs and Strays Society in 1890: 'I am sorry to tell you she has turned out very bad we found out last Sunday she had robbed us of money & articles from our shop.'

Although there is some acknowledgement in the case file of Maud's early experiences and the fact that her father and stepmother abused her, in line with dominant viewpoints of the time her behavioural issues are largely considered moral issues and problems, and the result of 'badness' (Maudsley, 1879; Sohasky, 2015). Yet, this view ignores the fact that behavioural issues can be a consequence of abuse and related mental health problems (Mash & Wolfe, 2019). Her 'being of a low moral type herself', using 'bad language' and 'behaving badly', being 'deceitful' and 'untruthful', seems to automatically classify Maud as 'undeserving' and beyond help, and to an extent reiterates the dominant focus on heredity of the time (Maudsley, 1879). This in and of itself seems to render her unworthy of support offered within the NSPCC (established in 1884) and the Prevention of Cruelty to and Protection of Children Act of 1889; the latter may be something Maud just missed out on.

During the late 1800s, whilst child philanthropy developed, providing child care services as an alternative to the workhouse, government welfare policy was focused on separating the 'deserving' from the 'undeserving', encouraging self-help and changing behaviour (Sohasky, 2015; Skinner & Thomas, 2017; Turner et al., 2015). It could be argued that, in this case, it was felt that Maud was a failure, unable to change her behaviour and immoral tendencies. Yet, the fact remains that, in judgements around deservedness, related stigmas around poverty and 'bad' behaviour are rife. This includes the danger of ignoring the link between child abuse and neglect and challenging behaviour, resulting in a situation where behaviour is inappropriately managed by punishing the child for their 'immoral tendencies' (Fisher et al., 2000; Hardwick, 2005). As such, it could be argued that Maud's case is an example of failure on the part of the COS, Poor Law authorities (Maud actually spent time in a workhouse as a small child) and the Waifs and Strays Society (Thane, 2012).

3.4 Janet (case file 9913): mentally deficient, thoroughly incompetent and unsatisfactory

Janet was born in 1894 in a mental asylum as an illegitimate child. She is looked after by her grandmother for a while, but ends up in a home for girls in 1905. A note from the doctor that year highlights that: 'I have this day examined Janet as to her mental condition. She seems to be somewhat dull in understanding, but she has no mental symptoms.' This seems to be in response to the observation that her mother is 'weak mentally', which highlights the dominant focus on heredity, in line with popular psychiatry/psychology of the time (see Rey et al., 2015). Between 1905 and 1909 Janet appears to have been moved from one home to another; for example, she finds herself in a home in Bristol in 1905 and one in Fareham in 1909 (117 miles apart). A letter from 1908 between the home Janet is in (it is not clear which home this is) and the Waifs and Strays Society indicates that 'she is not disobedient, but thoroughly incompetent'. In 1909, when Janet is 15, a letter appears from the home in Fareham saying:

I regret to inform you that the authorities of the Society's Fareham Home desire that she may be removed from their care as soon as arrangements can be made accordingly. Unfortunately in consequence of her mental deficiency and generally unsatisfactory physical condition, it has been found impossible to fit her for any place in service.

According to Henry Maudsley (1879), pioneering Victorian psychiatrist and founder of the eponymous mental hospital in London in 1907, a child cannot go 'mad', due to not having a mind to go wrong. Yet, this did not stop the authorities (in this case a children's home) from attaching the label of 'thoroughly incompetent' to Janet. Common diagnoses for those under the age of ten included 'idiocy' and 'imbecility', but did not necessarily indicate cognitive deficiencies (Sohasky, 2015; Rey et al., 2015).

In Chapter 1 I argued that, whilst on the surface 'the poor man/woman/child' (honest and industrious), 'the criminal' (disorderly and immoral) and 'the insane' (mentally ill) are not easy bedfellows, it is in the difficulty of and somewhat unwillingness to distinguish between the three that the ongoing influence of the deserving/undeserving paradigm can be seen in approaches to vulnerable children as their lives often overlapped in many ways. These were people (and their children) who walked the same paths between home, lodgings, unemployment, poor relief, charity and workhouse (Shore, 2003). This is also something that can be garnered from Janet's case, as her 'incompetence', 'mental deficiency' and 'unsatisfactory physical condition' – combined with her background of poverty and destitution – would have sealed her fate; and it is very likely that Janet ended up in the workhouse or an asylum after this.

3.5 Tracey (case file 4828): mental health issues (melancholia) and a burden

Tracey was born in 1892, and correspondence included in the application to the Waifs and Strays Society (dated 1895) highlights that: 'The mother has been in the asylum after the birth of most of the children and has since the birth of the last child, now two years ago, scarcely been able to be at home at all.' This suggests that Tracey's mother may have suffered from a postpartum psychiatric illness, also referred to as puerperal insanity, a term used extensively throughout the 19th century to describe mental illness following childbirth (Marland, 2004; Watts, 2011). The medical definition of puerperal insanity, combined with the ideal of motherhood as a purpose in life, allowed for a societal explanation for the 'strange' and 'odd' behaviour of mothers whilst at the same time ignoring power relationships in the family, social conditions and the material realities of mothering in this period (Campbell, 2017; Marland, 2012). In other words, puerperal insanity provided an explanation and 'justification' for some mothers' unusual behaviour after childbirth, ignoring the unequal social and material conditions that some women were exposed to. Moreover, the medical definition and inherent 'hereditary' nature of this 'burden' also reinforced the perception that various offspring could be (genetically) affected (Rey et al., 2015), as is discussed below. A letter from 1910 (when Tracey is 18) from the Old Town Hall Kennington (London) recordkeeper refers to the hereditary nature of the mother's mental health issues and the fact that she is in a lunatic asylum: 'It would seem that other members of the family are affected mentally, probably hereditary, and some of them are already a burden upon the father.'

It is apparent that Tracey is still in a home when she is 18 as a letter from the home to Edward Rudolf, founder of the Waifs and Strays Society, flags up her mental problems:

> As I have previously reported, this girl has lately behaved in a very strange manner and although since leaving her situation at Ardingley College, she has again had a trial in service, she made no effort in work, but spent most of her time in her bedroom.
>
> She was at one time a nice, industrious girl, but now is developing more and more unsatisfactory characteristics.
>
> She has been under the doctor and had medication, but it seems to be a case of melancholia.

References to the girl 'making no effort in work' and her 'unsatisfactory characteristics' are interesting in light of the notion of deservedness and how this was used by the Poor Law authorities to distinguish between people who were unable to work due to no fault of their own and those who were capable but unwilling, thereby undeserving of welfare support (Atherton, 2011; Skinner & Thomas, 2017). Although, this girl's mental health issues and her being 'a case of melancholia' would put her in the 'infirm' category, it is her accompanying lack of effort and unsatisfactory behaviour that appears to be centralised, rendering her undeserving here.

Among the correspondence is also a letter in 1909 from Tracey's mother saying that she has not seen her daughter for 12 months and had no reply to letters. She refers to 'married trouble that one cannot mention' and 'my mentale trouble has been through domestic troubles'. The latter hints at domestic violence, suggesting that the narrative around this mother and her children as a burden is very much a patriarchal one, favouring the father; this highlights the imbalance in family power relations and the dynamics of the time and in this family (Campbell, 2017; Watts, 2011).

The Victorian and Edwardian periods are intriguing areas for study due to various historical breakthroughs improving women's social, economic and domestic status, as well as attempts to curb domestic violence. Moreover, it was in the Victorian era that, for the first time in English history, specific standards were developed proclaiming the unacceptability of marital violence, which included the passing of acts and the establishment of institutions to aid victims (Moon, 2016). For example, the Society for the Prevention of Cruelty to Children (1884) and the Female Temporary Home (1852) were among places victims could go to escape domestic abuse (Moon, 2016); and in 1878 the UK Matrimonial Causes Act made it possible for women in the UK to seek legal separation from abusive husbands (Abrahams, 1999). The fact that Tracey's mother refers to 'domestic troubles' in her letter is perhaps a reflection of some of the progress that was made, putting women in a position where they felt they could speak out.

3.6 Jack (case file 9627): an imbecile and unsuitable for the home

The application for Jack's admittance to a Children's Home is dated 1903, when he is eight years old (born in 1895). His mother died of pneumonia and Jack's father is unable to look after his seven children. There is evidence that Jack is moved from home to home frequently, and the suggestion is that the homes are unable to cater to him; a letter, also from 1903, highlights this as follows:

> The boy, from all accounts, is not only quite helpless, but is also mentally deficient, and the strain, therefore, on the staff of the Home is such that I regret I must ask you to be good enough to have him removed without fail

and

> It is needless to say that I am always very grieved when the Society is obliged to relinquish the care of any child, but the fact unfortunately remains that there must be a certain number of children who are unsuitable for our Homes for some cause or other and the child in question is certainly one of them.

Interestingly, there are mixed messages in the correspondence around Jack – for example, various homes and institutions point to Jack's 'mental limitations' as a reason they cannot continue with him. For instance, Broadlands in Newport, Isle of Wight highlights in a letter that 'to hear that he is an imbecile is very sad' (1903), whilst in the same year there is a letter from Falmouth Hotel saying that 'his mental condition is not great'. This is in contrast to what is flagged up by a physician in a consultation: another letter from 1903 states that 'The doctor says he is a bright, intelligent child and he has great hopes for him.' What is not touched upon in most of the correspondence, apart from in the application, is that Jack is a 'cripple' due to polio.

In line with the deserving/undeserving paradigm, the 'infirm' were entitled to help and support as they found themselves in this position through no fault of their own, as opposed to being idle, lazy and workshy (Atherton, 2011; King, 2018). From this perspective Jack being a 'cripple' puts him in a position of entitlement and 'deservedness'. In this light it is quite interesting to see Jack's 'imbecility' and 'mental deficiency' being flagged as reasons he can no longer be supported by the children's homes. The fact that Jack's 'mental condition' puts a strain on the staff, whilst his physical condition is not referred to in this light, suggests that to an extent the onus is put on Jack to change this, as someone who is responsible for flaws in his mental ability but not his physical condition.

In line with the deserving/undeserving paradigm, there is a sense that Jack is being judged and held accountable for his behaviour, centralising self-responsibility and a need to change his behaviour (Sohasky, 2015; Skinner & Thomas, 2017; Turner et al., 2015). Moreover, the mixed messages around this, with the doctor describing Jack as bright and the various homes expressing regret about Jack's 'mental limitations', They also hint at confusion around the terms 'mental condition' and 'imbecility', and perhaps indicate that what is going on with Jack is not necessarily related to a cognitive deficiency but may be more behavioural. The decision to remove Jack from the home is not taken lightly, as can be seen above – this is encompassed by expressions of regret and grief. After all, in the greater scheme of things, the Waifs and Strays Society is relinquishing its duty to care for a destitute child by constructing Jack in terms of unsatisfactory and beyond help.

3.7 James (case file 16338): behavioural issues, 'fits of temper' and suicide

James was born in 1897, and his application is dated 1911 (when he is 14); at this time his mother is dead but his father is alive. In the application reference is made to the mother's demise and the fact that 'the children have all run very wild and become most unmanageable'. Interestingly, the blame for the children becoming unmanageable seems to be mostly put on James: 'The father cannot get anyone to stay as housekeeper, owing to this particular lad who is one of the greatest bullies and strikes the housekeepers and 'his language is filthy'.

From the date of the application onwards James seems to be in different homes and is moved to the Valley Hotel sometime between 1912 and 1914. In 1914 someone from Valley Hotel writes to the Waifs and Strays Society, saying that:

> I really cannot put up with him, he has such terrible fits of temper. Saturday he went out of the house saying he was going to drown himself, so I had to send one of my maids after him.

It continues:

> I have tried my best, but it is of no use, I don't think he can help himself.

Later in 1914, James drowns himself.

The unfortunate case of James is an example of the dangers implicit in considering emotional and behavioural problems as moral issues and problems, and something that is the result of 'badness' (e.g. the fact that James is apparently a bully) – ignoring the fact that behavioural issues can be a function of abuse and related mental health problems (Mash & Wolfe, 2019). It also again highlights the punitive nature of decisions based on 'deservedness': in this case the focus on behaviour and self-responsibility results in ignorance in relation to potential underlying problems and issues that James no doubt was suffering from, culminating in suicide.

3.8 Rose (case file 3469): 'uncontrollable' and 'unsatisfactory'

Rose was born in 1881 and her application appears when she is 11 years old, in 1892. There is not a lot of information about Rose's background, apart from the fact that she is an orphan and has 'defective hearing and eyesight'. In the application to the Waifs and Strays Rose is described as a nice girl who has had an unfortunate home life, as well as an illness: 'Rose is an exceedingly nice, good tempered child and has had a great deal to endure through the state of her home and through illness.'

There is evidence that Rose spends time in different homes and hospitals not run by the Waifs and Strays Society. In 1900 she ends up in the 'Clapham Home of Rest For Girls Out of Situation', and in the same year the following arrives in a letter at the Waifs and Strays Society: 'Rose conducted herself very unsatisfactory and has a violent temper, and was indeed so uncontrollable that at the last there was no alternative, but to place her in the workhouse.' This once more high-lights how 'bad behaviour' and a 'violent temper' are synonymous with 'undeservedness'; in this case it means that Rose is no longer perceived as eligible for help and support, and will be placed in the workhouse as a last resort (Atherton, 2011; Strand, 2016).

Again this negates the fact that, due to their pre-care experiences and potential trauma, looked after children may portray challenging emotional and behavioural difficulties (Fisher et al., 2000).This is in contrast with earlier communication acknowledging that Rose 'has had a great deal to endure'. It could be argued that the contrast between the earlier correspondence in relation to Rose being nice and good tempered and having had a great deal to endure and the later corre-spondence around her unsatisfactory behaviour highlights two poten-tial flaws of the time. First, it suggests that (as with the case files discussed earlier in this chapter) in the greater scheme of things, regardless of her potentially traumatic background, Rose is held accountable for her bad behaviour. Second, it shows that collabora-tions and communication between the various institutions/professionals was insufficient, and earlier experiences were not acknowledged. Included in the correspondence is also a letter from Rose of 1901:

> I am writing to ask you if you will allow me to go back to Clap-ham Home for I am really sorry for having to give so much trou-ble, I used to think that they were to strict but now I see that it was for my own good.

Despite the fact that there is reference to the girl's family history in the correspondence, and acknowledgement, to an extent, that she has had a very traumatic past, Rose's 'bad' behaviour takes centre stage. This approach is also adopted by Rose herself when she apologises for causing 'so much trouble'.

Thus, Rose's personal history of being in the care system and having had a great deal to endure, as well as her material context, places her on the margins of society with no privileges at all, something that is reflected in both Rose's correspondence and the correspondence of the professionals working with her.

3.9 Hannah (case file 7884): mental health issues, 'immoral tendencies' and 'impure talk'

Hannah is ten years old when she is taken on by the Waifs and Strays Society in 1900 after she is found wandering the streets. Both her parents are alive, but her mother is described as inebriated and the father is homeless, living in supported lodgings at times. Most of the correspondence (from Edward Rudolf as well as various homes and Hannah herself) is dated 1904, when Hannah is 14 years old; after this there is no communication until 1916. The final correspondence is dated 1931, when Hannah is 41. The first letter (dated April 1904) highlights that:

> Hannah is inclined to be very tiresome at present and was very much unsettled by the little play the children acted at Christmas. In fact, although it was beautifully acted I have greatly regretted having allowed it to take place. Hannah has always had a very wild look in her eyes as if her mind is not perhaps well-balanced and says and does the oddest things. She threatened to take her own life it may have been only bravado but she repeated this over and over again describing various methods by which suicide might be committed.

A further letter to Rudolf, also from April 1904, indicates that:

> I did quite right in taking the matter seriously and that in all probability there may be a family history, although from the casebook we are not able to discover this

and

> she has to be isolated at present, kept on low diet and the doctor has sent her some soothing medicine for the nerves. Hannah is very quiet and docile and has promised the doctor never to talk like that again.

However, it is clear that this is not the end of the matter, as a further letter to Rudolf arrives the same month, referring to 'the wildest kind of talk about suicide' and 'How, it is impurity of the very grossest kind, and such impure talk that unless we are very careful irremediable harm will be done to the children here, the details are so bad and revolting.'

Hannah is an example of the changing attitudes towards mental deficiency and insanity from the end of the 19th century, as part of which it became more widely acknowledged that juvenile insanity and 'madness' in children was different from mental retardation and epilepsy. Included in this was also recognition of the existence of suicide in children (Rey et al., 2015). At the same time, one couldn't quite escape the one-sided focus on physical causes and treatments, as can be seen from the talk about diet and medicine above. Moreover, the child rescue movement was very much driven by notions of morality (e.g. see Delap, 2015; Lynch, 2014; Sims-Schouten et al., 2019); and in this light suicide and related talk were perceived, as can be seen above (and underlined in the files), as 'impure' and 'revolting'. In July 1904 there is talk of charging Hannah under section 32 of the Industrial Schools Act 1866 and committing her to a Reformatory School. This prompts a letter from Edward Rudolf to the home in which he says:

> I notice that she [Hannah] has been in the Home since 1900 when she was ten years old and it seems strange she should now have become so very bad; I think the trouble you speak of should have been observed before.

This observation by Rudolf is interesting and shows an element of care and reflection. He acknowledges that Hannah has been in care since she was ten, and to an extent appears to question the care she has received so far and the inability of her carers to engage with her needs.

Our image of Victorian times is that of harsh care for children; think, for example, about the works by Charles Dickens. Moreover, research highlights how care in children's homes can also be seen in utter loneliness and lack of attention for children's needs (e.g. see Care of Children Committee, 1946). Yet, this is in contrast with other work which suggests that there is another side too. For example, Moss et al. (2017) researched child welfare and emigration institutions in 1870–1914, and argue that the image of the uncaring and emotionally distant institution does not reflect the ideology and practice of these (philanthropic) societies. As such, it is crucial to see this in light of different institutional, religious and philanthropic approaches of the time.

Reformatory Schools and Industrial Schools in Britain were established through the Reformatory Schools (Youthful Offenders) Act 1857 and the Industrial Schools Act 1857, consolidated in 1866 (Higginbotham, 2017). There was a key difference between reformatories and industrial schools, with the former catering for children who had committed a crime (and were perceived as in need of punishment) and the latter for children who had not yet committed a crime but were thought to be in circumstances that would make them likely to do so in the future (Cox, 2013). It should be noted, however, that by the end of the 19th century the roles had merged and it was impossible to easily tell the difference between the two.

Hannah was charged under the Industrial School Act and described as 'wilfully refusing to conform to the rules of the School'. Then, in October 1904, a letter appears from Hannah herself. In this letter of a couple of pages Hannah explains that she has been a naughty girl again for the last three days, but that the mistress has given her one more chance (and here she expresses her gratitude). She writes about going to church, going for walks and working in the mistress's kitchen. Moreover, she refers to a bad dream: 'I was very ill and at last I died, then I saw Satan and six of his angels standing ready for me.' A letter from the Industrial School follows in November 1905:

> We all feel that this girl requires hard work to take all the nonsense out of her. ... She is not an unmanageable girl, but one with strongly developed immoral tendencies and her temper is always cropping up.

Again, Hannah's immoral tendencies and behaviour appear to be at the forefront of the correspondence, which largely revolves around discussing how to manage, rather than support, her. There is no correspondence after this until 1916, a year which includes some letters from Hannah updating Edward Rudolf about her situation; here she mostly refers to her general illness and 'heart trouble'. There is also a letter in 1922 from a doctor referring to Hannah's general mental condition and her needing 'philanthropic friends', as well as indicating that she has a 'highly neurotic temperament'. The last letter regarding Hannah arrives in 1931, in which reference is made to her 'neurotic condition'.

3.10 Harry (case file 8645): a troubled past, an abusive system and a caring institution

Harry is another example of a young person who, like Hannah above, seems to have mixed experiences when it comes to the care provided by children's homes. Again, as discussed earlier, it would be too one-sided to refer to the (late) Victorian times in terms of a harsh and uncaring approach: as Moss et al. (2017) highlight, the image of the uncaring and emotionally distant institution does not reflect the ideology and practice of these (philanthropic) societies. Harry (born in 1893) is taken on by the Waifs and Strays Society in 1901 when he is eight years old; at this time all that is known is that his parents are both dead. In 1901 Harry ends up in Runwell Home (Essex), and in 1902 he writes a letter to Mrs W (the vicar's wife who was involved in Harry's admittance to Runwell) alleging cruel treatment at the home.

I am sorry I wrote that letter to Miss Wyley that I was happy, but I am not because one day I could not bend my legs and this is how he hit me, as he got a stick with bits of rope with nots on the ends and then he half killes us and we have to work all day the master will not let me stay in bed because I have a bad leg and could not walk but I had to go to school this is sad knews to here you must not say if you a letter say that i have writen this or eals he will kill me you must say that I shall have to come back you so I must be taken away from The Master and come to you and live with you and go to school there I am always crying to get away from him so I may close I remain your loving boy.

Mrs W expresses concern about this in a letter to Edward Rudolf: as can be seen from the extract below, she is taking the matter seriously and expresses concern about Harry's wellbeing (e.g. his unhappiness) and the treatment he may have received in the home.

I enclose you a letter from the little boy H – whom I sent to the Home at Runwell about 6 weeks ago. I must request you to enquire into it at once, for I cannot help feeling very anxious about him. I am also writing to my Brother-in-law Mr. J. The poor little fellow may be exaggerating – but he writes as though he was very unhappy & I shall not feel any confidence in the Master & shall probably decide to remove him. He has [?] hitherto had much discipline & I could fancy might in that account be troublesome but the roughest boy ought not to be treated so & if it is true, the sooner the House comes to an end the better. I shall be anxious to hear from you.

This account, to an extent, is evidence of the growing understanding and acknowledgement of the role of multiple factors in child wellbeing and behaviour at the time (e.g. see also Maudsley, 1879).

There is quite a bit of correspondence around this in which Edward Rudolf promises to look into the matter. In the same year (1902) a letter appears on behalf of Runwell Home and Reverend Harris:

Mr. Harris has asked me to write & tell you how very untruthful etc. we find H to be. … He has never been punished in any way since he has been here & the only work he has had to do is to help make the beds, but he is an extremely lazy boy & in the Cottage where he lived, evidently did just as he liked. It is only fair I think to us & our Master & Matron, that you should know these facts.

An investigation was carried out by Rudolf, part of which involved interviews with Harry and a Mr Jackson, who is associated with the home; in the end the story of the 'stick with knotted rope' is discounted as a fabrication. At the same time, Revd Edward Rudolf also notes that Harry continues to maintain that other boys had been told to hit him, and Rudolf felt there was possibly some truth in this. He asks the home to stop this practice at once (if it was happening), and reminds the staff of the correct procedure should a boy need to be punished. Below is a letter of 1902 from Rudolf to Reverend Harris providing his conclusions regarding Harry's complaints:

> I have questioned this boy and feel quite convinced that his statement respecting the stick with a knotted rope is sheer fabrication. He told me that he read a story before he came to the Home where one was mentioned, and that put it into his head, but he is evidently very untruthful, and it is just possible that he may have heard of such a stick in connection with the previous alleged cruelty. He stoutly maintains that the master told the other boys to hit him, and it is possible that there is some truth in this. If so, the practice should be at once stopped. Will you please make a careful enquiry on this point? When the boys require punishment, it must be administered by the master, and an entry made in the register. I return the letter which you were kind enough to send.

This information is passed on to Mrs W as well, whose response (by letter in 1902) is very much grounded in older traditions of morality and deservedness (Delap, 2015; Morrison, 2016), with a focus on moral improvement of the destitute. In other words, gone are her caring words and urge for better treatment; instead, she now requests punishment following Harry's deceit:

> I can't help feeling that if it is proved that he has not spoken the truth, he ought to be punished in some way or other [?] be bad for him to go in disgrace to a new school.

Nevertheless, shortly after this (also in 1902) Harry is moved to a different place, St Luke's Home for Boys in Sussex, and then in 1905 to St Benet's Home in Berkshire, where he thrives. St Benet's was particularly associated with gardening. In November 1907 the home's authorities write to Edward Rudolf telling him that they have received a request to discharge Harry to a woman in Alton (Hampshire) to learn cabinet making. They are not keen for him to go as "though not yet 15 years old, he is our best boy both in school and in [the] garden, and of great promise. I rather feel that he ought to rise, if properly assisted, above the rank of artisan." This plea, however, falls on deaf ears as Harry's brother is determined that Harry should take the opportunity that has arisen, to learn cabinet making, and the boy is discharged on 14 December 1907.

3.11 Annie (case file 7978): sexualised behaviour, immoral and impure

As with Harry discussed above, Annie's case also receives a mixed reception: on the one hand her early trauma and experiences are acknowledged as impacting upon her current behaviour, whilst at the same time her impurity and immorality are highlighted as matters of concern. Annie was found wandering the street in 1901 when she was 11 years old. Following this, she is taken into police custody and remanded on the charge of having no proper guardianship. Included in the correspondence is a letter from Salford Police Court (dated 1901) saying that: 'The girl's habits are bad, and she was the subject of an indecent assault, for which a man was tried and sentenced to penal servitude.'

Annie is taken on by a home in 1903, and there is talk of her 'trying to strangle herself' and 'having terrible fits': 'The girl, who I told you before was so troublesome and had several times tried to strangle herself.' Later in 1903 a letter is sent to the Waifs and Strays Society requesting her removal from the home due to her not being 'amenable to discipline'; a medical report at the same time refers to the girl as being a 'hysterical type'. There is also a letter from a vicarage in 1903 referring to her 'impure language':

> It is not childish naughtiness which one could understand and reason with, but a diseased mind, mostly owing to her miserable and ruined life in the past. Children pick up good and evil so quickly, it does seem wrong to let so much POISON get among them.

From the correspondence it is evident that Annie was the victim of an indecent assault. Here it is acknowledged that her 'miserable and ruined life in the past' was still influencing her, thereby recognising that there are multiple factors involved in the development of mental health issues in children (Rey et al., 2015). Included in this is reference to mental health issues, in the form of Annie being described as an 'hysterical type' – one of the first mental disorders specifically attributable to women and, until Freud, considered an exclusively female disease (Tasca et al., 2012). Yet, despite this and the fact that safeguarding measures were in place at the time (the NSPCC and the Prevention of Cruelty to and Protection of Children Act), in the final analysis Annie appears to be mainly measured against her behaviour and her 'diseased mind' and 'impure language', resulting in a request for her removal from the home. Authorities were concerned that girls who had been exposed to sexual behaviour would have a corrupting influence on other residents, and would remove them (Jackson, 1999; Wright & Digby, 1996).

3.12 Conclusion

The Victorian times were instrumental in instigating a number of changes to policy and practice with regard to safeguarding. For example, the Victorian era saw the establishment of a number of institutions and the introduction of Acts with a focus on child abuse and domestic abuse, such as the NSPCC (1884) and the Female Temporary Home (1852), where victims could go to escape domestic abuse (Moon, 2016). In 1878 the UK Matrimonial Causes Act made it possible for women in the UK to seek legal separation from abusive husbands (Abrahams, 1999).

Yet, the fact remains that children taken on by the Waifs and Strays Society were subject to judgement and confusion around their mental ability, related behaviour and deservedness, with the abuse and neglect that precedes this often overlooked. For example, in the cases discussed above Jack is described as both 'bright' and suffering from 'mental limitations', hinting at confusion around the term 'mental condition' and 'imbecility'. Annie appears to be mainly measured against her behaviour and her 'diseased mind' and 'impure language', resulting in a request for her removal from the home. Thus, what this chapter shows most of all is that, in the greater scheme of things, the Waifs and Strays Society was relinquishing its duty to care for the most vulnerable children and young people by constructing them in terms of beyond help – i.e. unsuitable, unmanageable, unsatisfactory, unfit and uncontrollable.

The data presented in this chapter highlights how the focus on individual accountability and responsibility in our current society strongly resembles the deserving/undeserving criteria promoted by the New Poor Law of 1834 and related harsh philosophy of self-care and self-responsibility (Sims-Schouten et al., 2019; Skinner & Thomas, 2017).

In judgements around 'deservedness', related stigmas around poverty and 'bad' behaviour are rife. Within this, the child's behaviour is inappropriately managed and the child is punished for his/her 'immoral tendencies', highlighting a need for more knowledge of and engagement with the underlying (psychological) reasons for their acute distress and abnormal behaviour (Fisher et al., 2000; Hardwick, 2005).

It is in this inability to distinguish 'the poor man/woman/child' (honest and industrious) from the 'the criminal' (disorderly and immoral) and 'the insane' (mentally ill) that the ongoing influence of the deserving/undeserving paradigm can be seen in approaches to vulnerable children as their lives often overlapped in many ways. Moreover, research highlights how care in children's homes can also be viewed as utter loneliness, which includes lack of attention for children's needs and trauma associated with neglect and abuse (e.g. see Care of Children Committee, 1946). At the same time, as Moss et al. (2017) argue, there is a need for balance as the image of the uncaring and emotionally distant (late) Victorian institutions does not always ring true, and it is crucial to see this in light of the different institutional, religious and philanthropic approaches of the time. This can be seen, for example, in the way in which Edward Rudolf questions the care provided to Hannah, which shows an element of care and reflection. Yet, what all the examples of cases presented in this chapter highlight is a need for a closer reflection on conceptualisations and 'realities' of 'problem children', mental health and child abuse and neglect, and the hidden pathways to resilience inherent in this (Ungar, 2002, 2004, 2005). The next chapter will provide an insight into the contemporary dataset, which consists of interviews with young care leavers and safeguarding practitioners.

Notes

1 See www.hiddenlives.org.uk and www.calmview.eu/childrensociety/Calm view/Record.aspx?src=CalmView.Catalog&id=TCS.
2 See www.hiddenlives.org.uk and www.calmview.eu/childrensociety/Calm view/Record.aspx?src=CalmView.Catalog&id=TCS.

References

Abrahams, L. (1999). Crime against marriage? Wife-beating, the law and divorce in nineteenth-century Hamburg. In: Arnot, M.L. and Usborne, C. (Eds.), *Gender and Crime in Modern Europe*. London: Routledge, 123–130.
Action for Children, NCB and Children's Society (2017). *Turning the Tide: Reversing the Move to Late Intervention Spending in Children and Young*

People's Services. https://www.childrenssociety.org.uk/sites/default/files/turning-the-tide.pdf.

Atherton, M. (2011). Deserving of charity or deserving of better? The continuing legacy of the 1834 Poor Law Amendment Act for Britain's deaf population. *Review of Disability Studies,* 7(3–4), 18–25.

Bazalgette, L., Rahilly, T. and Trevelyan, G. (2015). *Achieving Emotional Wellbeing for Looked After Children: A Whole System Approach.* London: NSPCC. https://learning.nspcc.org.uk/media/1122/achieving-emotional-wellbeing-for-looked-after-children.pdf.

Bhaskar, R. (2014). Foreword. In: Edwards, P., O.Mahoney, J. and Vincent, S. (Eds.), *Studying Organizations Using Critical Realism: A Practical Guide.* Oxford: Oxford University Press, v–xv.

Campbell, M.A. (2017). 'Noisy, restless and incoherent': puerperal insanity at Dundee Lunatic Asylum. *History of Psychiatry,* 28(1), 44–57.

Care of Children Committee (1946). *Report of the Care of Children Committee.* London: HMSO.

Cox, P. (2013). *Bad Girls in Britain: Gender, Justice and Welfare, 1900–1950.* Basingstoke: Palgrave Macmillan.

Delap, L. (2015). Child welfare, child protection and sexual abuse, 1918–1990, *History & Policy.* http://www.historyandpolicy.org/policy-papers/papers/child-welfare-child-protection-and-sexual-abuse-1918-1990.

Fisher, T., Gibbs, I., Sinclair, I. and Wilson, K. (2000). Sharing the care: the qualities sought of social workers by foster carers. *Child & Family Social Work,* 5(3), 225–233.

Gingell, K. (2001). The forgotten children: children admitted to a county asylum between 1854 and 1900. *Psychiatric Bulletin,* 25, 432–434.

Hacking, I. (1991). The making and molding of child abuse. *Critical Inquiry,* 17(2), 253–288.

Hardwick, L. (2005). Fostering children with sexualised behaviour. *Adoption & Fostering,* 29(2), 33–43.

Higginbotham, P. (2017). *Children's Homes. A History of Institutional Care for Britain's Young.* Barnsley: Pen & Sword History.

Jackson, L.A. (1999). *Child Sexual Abuse in Victorian England.* London: Routledge.

King, S.A. (2018). *Sickness, Medical Welfare and the English Poor, 1750–1834.* Manchester: Manchester University Press.

Lynch, G. (2014). Saving the child for the sake of the nation: moral framing and the civic, moral and religious redemption of children. *American Journal of Cultural Sociology,* 2, 165–196. doi:10.1057/ajcs.2014.5.

Marland, H. (2004). *Dangerous Motherhood: Insanity and Childbirth in Victorian Britain.* Basingstoke: Palgrave Macmillan.

Marland, H. (2012). Under the shadow of maternity: birth, death and puerperal insanity in Victorian Britain. *History of Psychiatry,* 23(1), 78–90.

Mash, E. and Wolfe, D. (2019). *Abnormal Child Psychology.* Belmont, CA: Wadsworth.

Maudsley, H. (1879). *The Pathology of Mind.* London: Macmillan.

Melling, J., Adair, R. and Forsythe, B. (1997). 'A proper lunatic for two years': pauper lunatic children in Victorian and Edwardian England. Child admissions to the Devon County Asylum, 1845–1914. *Journal of Social History,* 31(2), 371–394.

Moon, J. (2016). *Domestic Violence in Victorian and Edwardian Fiction.* Newcastle upon Tyne: Cambridge Scholars.

Morrison, J. (2016). *Familiar Strangers, Juvenile Panics and the British Press: The Decline of Social Trust.* London: Palgrave Macmillan.

Moss, E., Wildman, C., Lamont, R. and Kelly, L. (2017). Rethinking child welfare and emigration institutions, 1870–1014. *Cultural and Social History,* 14(5), 647–668.

Rey, J.M., Assumpção, F.B., Bernad, C.A., Çuhadaroğlu, F.C., Evans, B., Fung, D., Harper, G., Loidreau, L., Ono, Y., Pūras, D., Remschmidt, H., Robertson, B., Rusakoskaya, O.A. and Schleimer, K. (2015). History of child and adolescent psychiatry. In: Rey, J.M. (Ed.), *IACAPAP e-Textbook of Child and Adolescent Mental Health.* Geneva: International Association for Child and Adolescent Psychiatry and Allied Professions, 1–67.

Sampson, O.C. (1976). Treatment practices in British child guidance clinics: an historical overview. *Educational Review,* 29(1), 13–29.

Shore, H. (2003). Crime, criminal networks and the survival strategies of the poor in early eighteenth-century London. In: King, S. and Tomkins, A. (Eds.), *The Poor in England, 1700–1850.* Manchester and New York: Manchester University Press, 137–165.

Sims-Schouten, W., Skinner, A. and Rivett, K. (2019). Child safeguarding in light of the deserving/undeserving paradigm: a historical and contemporary analysis. *Child Abuse & Neglect,* 94. doi:10.1016/j.chiabu.2019.104025.

Skinner, A. and Thomas, N. (2018), 'A pest to society': the Charity Organisation Society's domiciliary assessments into the circumstances of poor families and children. *Children & Society, 32,* 133–144. doi:10.1111/chso.12237.

Sohasky, K.E. (2015). Safeguarding the interests of the state from defective delinquent girls. *Journal of the History of Behavioral Sciences, 52*(1), 20–40. doi:10.1002/jhbs.21765.

Stein, M. (2006). Research review: young people leaving care. *Child and Family Social Work,* 11(3), 273–279.

Stewart, J. (2011). 'The dangerous age of childhood': child guidance and the 'normal' child in Great Britain, 1920–1950. *Paedagogica Historica,* 47, 785–803.

Strand, M. (2016). Historicizing social inequality: a Victorian archive for contemporary moral discourse. *American Journal of Cultural Sociology,* 5(1–2), 225–260.

Tasca, C., Rapetti, M., Carta, M.G. and Fadda, B. (2012). Women and hysteria in the history of mental health. *Clinical Practice & Epidemiology in Mental Health,* 8, 110–119. doi:10.2174/1745017901208010110.

Thane, P. (2012). The 'big society' and the 'big state': creative tension or crowding out? *Twentieth Century British History,* 23, 408–429.

Turner, J., Hayward, R., Angel, K., Fulford, B., Hall, J., Millard, C. and Thomson, M. (2015). The history of mental health services in modern England: practitioner memories and the direction of future research. *Medical History*, 59(4), 599–624. doi:10.1017/mdh.2015.48.

Ungar, M. (2004). *Nurturing Hidden Resilience in Troubled Youth*. Toronto: University of Toronto Press.

Ungar, M. (2005). *A Handbook for Working with Children and Youth: Pathways to Resilience across Cultures and Contexts*. Thousand Oaks, CA: Sage.

Ungar, M. (2002). *Playing at Being Bad: The Hidden Resilience of Troubled Teens*. Halifax, NS: Pottersfield Press.

Vaismoradi, M., Turunen, H. and Bondas, T. (2013). Content analysis and thematic analysis: implications for conducting a qualitative descriptive study. *Nursing & Health Sciences*, 15, 398–405.

Ward, H. (1990). *The Charitable Relationship: Parents, Children and the Waifs and Strays Society*. PhD thesis, University of Bristol. https://research-information.bristol.ac.uk/files/34489504/292443.pdf.

Watts, A. (2011). 'Mother's interrupted: puerperal insanity in early twentieth century Australia', paper presented to Mothers at the Margins, Sixth International Conference on Motherhood, University of Queensland, Brisbane, 27–30 April.

Wright, D. and Digby, A. (Eds.) (1996). *From Idiocy to Mental Deficiency: Historical Perspectives on People with Learning Disabilities*. London and New York: Routledge.

4 The case of care leavers, mental health and safeguarding in contemporary Britain

In this chapter, I will put the experiences of young care leavers in contemporary Britain into perspective, drawing on the voice of the most vulnerable care leavers, referred to by Stein (2006) as 'victims'. From the 1970s onwards research has highlighted the adversities faced by children and young people leaving the care system (e.g. see Stein & Carey, 1986). Currently, whilst there is considerable quantitative data around the circumstances of care leavers in the UK, there is still little qualitative research with a focus on their experiences and perceptions. Similarly, there is little research that draws attention to practitioner experiences and perceptions; as it stands, care-leaving programmes, projects and support are generally more focused on education, employment and housing issues than on addressing the mental health and wellbeing needs of young people (Sims-Schouten & Hayden, 2017).

Care leavers are the group of young people who have spent time in care and/or have grown up in the care system and find themselves in the position of having to leave the care system (whether they are ready or not), either to become independent or with some form of ongoing support – e.g. in the form of after-care, ongoing support from social work and/or counselling (Coman & Devaney, 2011; Eronen, 2011). Definitions and perceptions of who can be classified as a care leaver have, however, varied over the decades. Following the Children (Leaving Care) Act 2000, a child is defined as a 'care leaver' if they are aged 16 or 17 and have been looked after by a local authority for a period of 13 weeks, starting after the age of 14 and ending at 16 (Community Care, 2001; DfE, 2015). Moreover, minors generally 'cease to be looked after' at age 18 (Sims-Schouten & Hayden, 2017). It should also be noted that some prefer the term 'care-experienced' over 'care leaver' or 'looked after child'; 'care-experienced' refers to anyone who has been, or is currently, in care.

Care leavers comprise only a small minority of the total population of young people in the UK; roughly 90,000 children pass through the care system each year, and around 30,000 cease to be 'looked after' (DfE, 2015; Sims-Schouten & Hayden, 2017). Currently, local authorities are bound by the 'staying put' duty implemented by the Children and Families Act 2014, meaning that young care leavers are entitled to continued support and living arrangements once they turn 18 (DfE, 2015; Lindsay, 2014). It is well evidenced that care leavers, as a group, experience higher levels of unemployment and homelessness, and are more likely to be teenage parents compared to other groups of young people: they also have more disabilities, lack formal qualifications and are over-represented in the prison population (Richardson & Lelliott, 2003). Moreover, according to the World Health Organization, unemployment, homelessness and imprisonment are known to intersect with higher levels of mental health problems (WHO, 2012). Yet, the links between mental health and wellbeing and pre-care experiences are complex and varied, and experiences whilst in care and of leaving care add to this complexity (Akister et al., 2010; Dixon, 2008; Paul et al., 2015; Stein & Dumaret, 2011). As with the previous chapter, drawing on critical realist ontology and thematic content analysis, this chapter will shed light on this complexity.

4.1 Care leavers: mental health issues, behaviour and complex needs

As with Chapter 3, the current chapter focuses on young people with complex (mental health) needs and damaging pre-care, care and post-care experiences, referred to by Mike Stein (2006) as 'victims'. Unlike the care leavers groups defined by Stein as the 'moving on' group and the 'survivor' group, the 'victim' group are the most disadvantaged. After leaving care they are likely to be unemployed and to become homeless, to be lonely and isolated and to have mental health problems. The contemporary dataset used here consists of interviews with both care leavers who fit the 'victim' category and safeguarding practitioners/ professionals. A total of 46 participants were interviewed, 24 young care leavers and 22 safeguarding practitioners (care workers, family services managers, safeguarding officers in schools and safe guarding managers); all participants came from urban areas in South-East England. Of the 24 young people who took part in the interviews, 11 were male and 13 female; 7 of the participants were from a black, Asian and minority ethnic (BAME) background (2 males, 4 females). Note that, in comparison, the participants in the historic dataset were all Caucasian. The average age of the participants was 18.5 years, with the youngest 17 and the oldest 22; on average they had spent ten years in care. All participants were living in supported accommodation at the time of the interview, and all had an unstable care trajectory in line with Stein's definition of 'victims'. Of all the young people, 12 were in education (college), 4 were employed and 8 were not in education or employment.

The 22 safeguarding practitioners (2 men and 20 women; one from a BAME background) comprised: 8 care workers linked to family support charities and children's charities catering for children in care, careleavers and vulnerable families; 3 family services managers; 3 service leads for young people's support and housing; 4 safeguarding officers linked to 3 secondary schools; 2 community care workers; and 2 managers of a family centre. Data protection rules were followed, ethical consent was obtained for the interviews, and the research was reviewed and approved by the University Ethics Committee. See Table 4.1 for participant information.

As with the historic dataset, data collection focused on a number of key topics – including mental health, wellbeing, needs and behaviour – and data was collected through (individual) semi-structured interviews with the young care leavers and safeguarding professionals. Data collection and analysis was grounded in and informed by the three-phased critical realist analysis introduced in Chapter 2; this will be discussed in more detail in the next section.

Table 4.1 Summary of participant information

	Care leaver group	Practitioner group
Average time in care	10 years (ages 6–15)	Not known
Profession/education	In education, N=12 In employment, N=4 Not in education or employment, N=8	After-care worker: N=8 safeguarding officer (school): N=4 Service lead for support and housing: N=3 Family service manager: N=3 Community care worker: N=2 Family centre manager: N=2
Gender	Female, N=13; male N=11	Female, N=20; male, N=2
Ethnicity	BAME, N=7 (5 female; 2 male)	BAME, N=1 (female)

4.2 Institutional/organisational factors, social policy/social work and psychology/psychiatry

As with the historic dataset in Chapter 3, phase 1 comprised a thorough and focused review of relevant literature, policy documents, secondary data and grey literature to identify the most common elements of embodiment, institutions and materiality that (may) impact the participants. Table 4.2 summarises the outcome of phase 1 of the study, and provides examples of psychological and political structures and institutions as well as contextual factors in relation to care leavers in

Table 4.2 Institutions/organisations, social policy/social work and psychology/psychiatry factors: dataset 2 – care leavers and safeguarding practitioners/professionals (2015–2017)

Institution/organisation	Social policy/social work	Psychology/psychiatry
Responsibility for providing services for care-experienced children and young people (e.g. mental health and safeguarding) lies with local authorities, social care and the voluntary sector Children's Society, and Care Leavers Association: examples of charities delivering services for children in care and young care leavers 'Staying put' and 'staying in touch' duty: local authorities must provide/ensure living arrangements for children/young people in care once they turn 18 and monitor progress on their pathway plans (Children and Families Act, 2014)	Working Together to Safeguard Children legislation (2015): statutory guidance on inter-agency working to safeguard and promote the welfare of children Children and Social Work Act (2017), implemented to improve safeguarding, welfare and multiagency working Council spending on early intervention services designed to spot signs of abuse and neglect cut by 40% between 2010/11 and 2014/15 Cuts to children's services (2010/11–2016/17); services in the South cut by 23%	Focus on the role of multiple factors (social, psychological, biological) in mental health and mental health issues in childhood Transition from Child and Adolescent Mental Health Services (CAMHS) to adult mental health services

Sources: Action for Children et al., 2017, 2018; DfE, 2015; NSPCC, 2016; Rey et al., 2015.

England (but note that it is by no means exhaustive). In line with critical realist ontology and epistemology, these factors are treated as non-linear dynamics and generative mechanisms that may or may not be activated, depending on conditions.

Phase 1 informed the data collection tool: in this case we used semi-structured interviews as well as additional measures – namely observational methods and existing relevant data (e.g. on local mental health provision) – to create a factsheet for each participant to record material, institutional and embodied conditions that may have affected their experiences (see also Sims-Schouten & Riley, 2018).

Phase 2 of the three-phase analysis comprises thematic content analysis of the semi-structured interviews in order to identify themes, patterns and contrasts across the datasets. A number of key themes were identified across both datasets – the details relating to the contemporary dataset are summarised in Table 4.3.

Table 4.3 Talk about and by the young person

Themes	Interviews with safeguarding practitioners, N=22	Interviews with care leavers, N=24
'Beyond help' (not wanting to be helped; no purpose; criminal children)	50% (N=10)	–
'Centralising the needs of the child'	50% (N=11)	–
'Mental health issues' (a problematic child)	46% (N=10)	42% (N=10)
'Behavioural issues' (a problematic child)	28% (N=6)	29% (N=7)
Mental health issues & behavioural issues both mentioned	23% (N=5)	17% (N=4)
Child abuse & neglect	54% (N=12)	22% (N=5); NB: this is mostly about neglect by the state as the corporate parent and neglect in care
Sexual abuse/sexualised behaviour	14% (N=3)	–
'Grateful'	–	63% (N=15)
I am/used to be 'bad'	–	42% (N=10)

In line with critical realist ontology, the final phase was used to identify links between how the participants make sense of themselves and the wider institutional discourses producing some of the conditions enabling this sense-making. This involved examining the data in terms of how participants' personal, material and institutional contexts may have affected their experiences. Below I will discuss and analyse examples of the responses of both care leavers and safeguarding practitioners in light of the themes outlined in Table 4.3. As in Chapter 3, pseudonyms are used in order to protect the participants' identities.

4.3 Aaron: mental health and behavioural issues – 'we shouldn't be dealing with this'

Aaron is 22 years old and has been in the care system (foster care and children's homes) since he was three. His father is estranged from the family and his mother, who died when Aaron was 19, had a history of mental health issues. Currently, Aaron receives support from an after-care charity and lives in supported accommodation with his partner and baby daughter. Between the ages of 16 and 18 Aaron was homeless and lived on the street; he also received a suspended jail sentence during this time for threatening a shop assistant. Below are extracts from the interview with Aaron, as well as the after-care charity and a worker at the hostel where Aaron spent time when he was 18. Aaron suffers from depression and anxiety, but apart from the after-care charity is receiving limited support through counselling services. Here Aaron is reflecting on his experience in the care system:

> I can only use a term that I've been a hard-nosed bastard all my life, umm if you grow up in the care system then there is not much that can scare you, there is not much that can you know what I mean put fear into you. The most scariest thing I've done in my life, you know what I mean is watch my little girl be born. Hmm that is the most scariest thing. I mean losing my Mum was upsetting but it happens you know what I mean. When you're in that system. Where you've got a parental figure and you've got nothing like that and people say they're your parental figure and don't actually help you.

In this extract Aaron is referring to what is known as the 'corporate parenting' role of local authorities. This infers that local authorities have to act as the best possible parent for each child they look after, which includes acting as advocate on the child/young person's behalf to secure the best possible outcomes (DfE, 2015).

Specialist services for care leavers developed in the 1980s, with a specific focus on education and support with practical skills (Stein and Carey, 1986). Moreover, since the implementation of the Children (Leaving Care) Act 2000 in England and Wales and the 'corporate parenting model', responsibility for young care leavers rests with a case worker or 'personal advisor', who works with other agencies regarding issues around accommodation, education, employment and training (Community Care, 2001; Stein, 2006). Yet, as can be seen from Aaron's experience, the corporate parent can be less than satisfactory, and more can be done to help vulnerable young people with their mental health and wellbeing (see also Sims-Schouten & Hayden, 2017):

> I haven't had many people in my life who will just be there. Like I can argue that my mum was there for me, but she wasn't there for me if that makes sense, because I have one older brother, two younger and two younger sisters so she had to also be there for them. And I weren't in the family, in the family. It was easier for her to be there for them than it was for me but then I'd had a social worker who'd said that she was there for me but whenever I had a problem and turned around to her and said look these are my problems. She'd be like 'oh I can't help you. I've got a thousand other cases. You are not that important you are doing fine!' kind of thing. And then they palmed me off somewhere else. They just said: 'look, don't come to us anymore, use your new support worker'. Because it got to a point where I was being physically and verbally violent towards them.

The discussion above suggests that in Aaron's perception of the lack of care he received there is a sense of what is known as 'passing the buck' (see also Steffel et al., 2016). Research highlights that in multi-agency contexts there is a tendency to pass the buck when there is a perceived risk of being held accountable and/or possibly blamed for a bad outcome (e.g. see Morrison, 2016; Steffel et al., 2016). By linking this to being 'physically and verbally violent towards them' there is also a sense of a punitive element (Hardwick, 2005; Holland, 2000; Waechter et al., 2019). The focus here is on a reductionist or isolated notion of the individual (i.e. the bad behaviour) rather than larger-scale social structures (e.g. issues around care and provision) (Dagnan, 2007; Toms, 2012). To this effect, Stein (2008) has highlighted the importance of promoting resilience in care leavers, applying the personal advisor concept to wider aspects of care and leaving care experiences. However, it is also important to acknowledge hidden pathways to resilience, and Aaron's 'disordered behaviour' may be the only strategy available to him in light of being passed from pillar to post (Ungar, 2002, 2004, 2005).

Below are some of the reflections of the after-care charity worker in Aaron's case:

> And then we have XXplus which is our properties, like a supported housing scheme. So we can have up to ten flats and ... the young people have to have been a part of this. From the beginning. They have to be, have had a go in the flat. Erm and they have to, are meant to have been in employment or education and then it is for young people who are in the life-skills programme but they haven't got any other alternative accommodation opportunity for them. So it might be that they've been in other housing and support, but they've been evicted and so they won't have them back or maybe they've had a bit of anti-social behaviour ... or for whatever reason, they can't get an alternative accommodation situation and they've come to the end of either their children's home or their foster care placement.

This extract further evidences the ongoing influence of the deserving/undeserving paradigm as, although help is offered through the supported housing scheme, it is also made clear that this is only available to those who have been in employment or education. This shows how the notion of deservedness has fed into the creation of the welfare state as an insurance-based system, with a clear relationship between paying your dues and deserving help (see also Shah & Cook, 2008). Here entitlement can be directly aligned with the workings of the Poor Law, i.e. those who work and/or are in education are deserving of supported housing (Atherton, 2011; King, 2019).

This is also interesting in light of the latter part of the extract, where reference is made to anti-social behaviour as a reason those young people may have been evicted from other accommodation/support; this seems a bit of a contrast when seen in light of the requirement to be in employment or education. In other words, the fact that the supported accommodation facilities are only provided to young people who are in education and/or employment may rule out a number of more vulnerable young people – those who, due to complex problems and behavioural, have either been evicted from accommodation or not been in a position to consistently embark on either education or employment. Yet, the blame seems to be with them. As such, there is ignorance of the correlation between certain 'bad' behaviours and an abusive past.

The following extract comes from a service lead worker in a hostel that Aaron was evicted from due to anti-social and aggressive behaviour:

> Our connections are very strong with some of those agencies. So, with the Council, especially like housing departments, social care, very very strong, very tight, the way that we work, and not too bad with criminal justice systems, health services, physical health, doctors are usually quite good, mental health services have always been the tricky one, for us. Cause we have residents who aren't always mentally very well and when their mental health deteriorates and we can see a problem we're looking for support that isn't always there. And then we're left as untrained, we're not trained mental health practitioners, we shouldn't be dealing with this, the sort of mental health issues that we are sometimes.

This highlights that, when it comes to child safeguarding, protection and mental health support, there continues to be a complex mix of teams involved, sometimes with evidence of poor integration of welfare, mental health services and social care (Frost et al., 2005; Priest et al., 2011). As the service lead above says, 'mental health services have always been the tricky one for us'. Aaron has a history of mental health issues and trauma, sometimes resulting in aggressive behaviour when he feels that his needs are not being catered to. By referring to not being trained mental health practitioners, the agency above is once again passing the buck.

4.4 John: behavioural issues, getting angry and needing to control his emotions

John has been in care since he was at primary school, mostly children's homes; he has mild learning difficulties and currently lives in a support home for young adults (aged 18–25). He is very keen to move into supported accommodation, and in the interview he appears very angry about having to wait for this. This can also be seen in the following short extract from the interview, which is part of a discussion around the fact that he had expected to move to supported accommodation in January (the interview took place in April):

JOHN: I had some issues on the way as well. Uhhh ... it just feels like to me: 'Oh, I'm going in January then I've got to go home and then I've got to wait'. It is a bit like, it is just too long and I don't wanna wait that long.

WENDY: So you are not sure whether you are staying where you are now for a while?

JOHN: Yeah. I JUST DON'T LIKE IT TO BE HONEST, BUT NOTHING I CAN DO.

In the interview John repeatedly refers to his anger issues, and also explains that he has been evicted from a number of schools because of this. Currently he receives support from different agencies – an after-case charity and children's charity, as well as social workers. He is reflecting on some of this below:

JOHN: Uhh they've like it's helped me with like emotion skills a bit better.

WENDY: Yeah? What have you learnt on this front?

JOHN: Umm doing different things to stop getting angry. I still get angry and need to work out what the thing is and if they're doing it, but it's helped like a little bit not a lot but a little bit.

Again, John's bad behaviour takes centre stage here, rather than larger-scale social structures such as the fact that supported accommodation is not yet forthcoming for him (Dagnan, 2007; Toms, 2012). In his account this translates into a reflection on his individual flaws, emotions and behaviour, rather than the dynamics in the immediate social context – essentially locating 'problems' (emotional and behavioural issues) in the individual, who is held accountable (Skinner & Thomas, 2018).

John has been expelled from a number of schools, and although he has settled in reasonably well in the college he is currently attending, it is clear that the onus is on him, with a focus on self-responsibility, self-help and changing his behaviour (Sohasky, 2015; Skinner & Thomas, 2018; Turner et al., 2015).

Below is an extract from an interview with the deputy head/safeguarding officer in a school for children with behavioural, emotional and social difficulties.[1] In the interview she reflects on the fact that some children are uncontrollable and beyond help (as they are 'criminal children'), again placing the responsibility to behave properly with the child:

Because we've had quite a few cases, like I was saying, where staff are assaulted, or there's huge amounts of criminal damage. And where there's this policy about not criminalising children, that actually is quite hard for us to get our heads around, because, well we are a social, emotional and mental health school, so we have pretty much the naughtiest children in the city and whilst I understand that a good kid who does one bad thing is not a criminal, we have one young person who has had ninety-one criminal offences. And that's a way beyond a good kid doing one thing bad, sometimes these are criminal children doing criminal activities repeatedly, repeatedly, repeatedly, and at that, at some point, restorative is not good enough, it's not working.

In this extract a direct link is made between being a 'social, emotional and mental health school' and working with 'the naughtiest children in the city'. Within this though, the young person is held accountable and construed as criminal (i.e. 'undeserving'). The extract refers to 'restorative' practice, which is widely used in school settings and practices in England as a way to work through, resolve and transform conflicts (Zehr, 2015). Yet, in this case, it is felt, as evidenced in the discussion above, that some children are beyond help on this front.

4.5 Katie: mental health, stress, upset and needing someone to talk to

Katie is originally from the Gambia, and little is known about her early childhood; she moved to the UK when she was 13 years old and has been in care ever since. Katie is currently 20, and her time in the UK has been fraught with issues around bullying, racist incidents and mental health problems (anxiety and stress). She currently lives in supported accommodation, which was organised by her social worker, and she receives help from an after-care charity.

Below Katie talks about her specific needs and what help and support she feels she could benefit from:

> I was struggling with money, and sometimes I have nobody to talk to and stuff. I am getting so much stress that my hair is falling out, and it is so hard to handle, you know. I need someone that I can talk to, so I can talk to them and that can make me feel better, like when I am upset.

> I was getting into debt, which was just me being silly basically. I was just like, erm because when I get really upset, I had to do shopping. Shopping helped me.

> They think that I'm all grown up, but it doesn't work like that.

> I am not feeling well as I haven't been eating so.

> Yeah, because, for me, I don't know. I am a good tempered person. So, basically for me, if somebody will talk to me and that's someone I don't get on with really really easily, then.

It could be argued that Katie is a victim of changing thresholds for support, which should be seen in light of ongoing cuts to support and services (Action for Children et al., 2017, 2018). This is evident from her saying that 'they think I'm all grown up, but it doesn't work like that'. Although Katie is 20 years old, it is clear that she is still in need of support, for example in relation to her mental health and wellbeing (she is stressed and upset); yet support appears variable. There is evidence of age, socioeconomic and ethnic inequality in NHS provision, creating new stratifications of exclusion and inclusion (Jørgensen & Thomsen, 2018; Shah & Cook, 2008). It could be argued that this goes hand in hand with a renewed focus on individual accountability and responsibility, which strongly resembles the deserving/undeserving criteria introduced by the Poor Law of 1834.

The following extract comes from an interview with an after-care worker who reflects on the help (or lack of help) available, and the fact that some of the support stops when young people turn 18. This interviewee works for the after-care charity that caters for Katie's supported accommodation and also provides a 'life-skills' programme as part of this (see also Sims-Schouten & Hayden, 2017):

> The main issues are money and accommodation, but also mental wellbeing is a massive factor that affects everything, I think. And what I have noticed with these young people is that they don't always want to discuss their mental health, because they see it as a stigma. I mean I don't think it is as much as what it used to be, because it is more in the media now isn't it, and a lot more people are talking about it. And a lot of our young people, on their referral forms it might say: 'any mental health needs?' And if it says yes – usually it's because of, obviously the way they've been bought up or what's happened to them, if they were mainly left on their own, or that they don't know their parents, they haven't got a good connection with their family – because of that: they have also had work with CAMHS, the child and adolescent mental health service.
>
> The issue with that though is that when they turn eighteen – that support stops. That's a massive problem and I think because it stops at eighteen a lot of the young people think, 'oh well, I don't have to worry about it now'. And I wonder if it is, when they are older, it might be then that they might reflect a bit and think actually, I needed some help with my mental health. I think that, when they are eighteen maybe between eighteen and twenty two; they don't see it as an issue. Although their mental health does

affect their everyday life. Some young people don't wanna be in groups, some young people who are not in education, don't wanna go to college because they don't like being in massive groups of people. Where that stems from could be to do with a multitude of things, you know I'm not a mental health practitioner but I try to listen to them to understand. Because you can't force someone to go to college and do a course if they don't want to do it, d'you know. So I would say, money, mental health and accommodation are the main three, I'd say, the main issues. Yeah.

This after-care worker acknowledges that mental health 'is a massive factor that affects everything', whilst also referring to issues around transitioning from child and adolescent mental health services to adult mental health support, and the changing thresholds there (the issue being that when they turn 18 the support stops). Research highlights that transitioning from child and adolescent mental health services (CAMHS) to adult mental health services (AMHS) can be proble-matic, and often young people with mental health problems find themselves without professional support or a referral to an adult ser-vice, or are referred to adult services that are ill-equipped to meet their needs (see Hood, 2016; Sims-Schouten & Hayden, 2017; Winter, 2014). Moreover, use of mental health services in the UK and the USA declines drastically when young people reach 16 years of age (by 24 and 45 per cent, respectively), and even more so at the age of 18 (over 60 per cent in the UK) (Singh & Tuomainen, 2015). This is due to changing thresholds and transition difficulties, with young people who have emotional/neurotic and personality disorders reporting as having more pronounced transition difficulties (Paul et al., 2015; Singh & Tuomainen, 2015; Winter 2014).

4.6 Claire: mental health issues, low confidence and 'keeping everything calm'

Claire is 17 years old and has been in and out of care for a large part of her life. She has three sisters (one of whom is a half-sister); she lives with her younger sister in foster care. Claire is supported by a complex team of carers, from social workers to mental health support workers, and she is now also supported by an after-care charity due to her soon becoming a care leaver when she turns 18. As mentioned in Chapter 1, when it comes to child safeguarding, protection and mental health support there continues to be a complex mix of teams involved, with evidence of poor integration of welfare, mental health services and social care (Frost et al., 2005; Priest et al., 2011). This is also evident from discussions with Claire:

> It's like, new people, I don't really get on with new people. I am always being introduced to new people, constantly, and then I have to tell my story again. All the social workers I've had pretty much never appreciated it so. I'm hoping to get my old social worker back soon

At the same time, there is a sense that Claire needs the mix of support that she receives, and to an extent she also benefits from this: 'Cause I get quite stressed at home, quite a lot so my social worker got X [mental health project] involved to help me with that.'

With regard to her mental health and wellbeing, Claire states: 'I do get some support with it, like they give me ideas as well and X shows how to keep everything calm.' Moreover, when asked if the support she is getting has helped her mental health and wellbeing, she says: 'It was mainly my confidence when talking to other people, with like, business like banks, doctors, people like that. I never really had confidence to do it', but also: 'I've got my social worker and foster parents, and X, so am getting a lot of support from everywhere.'

Towards the end of the interview the discussion revolves around leaving care, and Claire highlights that, although she has been involved in a number of support groups, 'I don't get involved in that anymore, because I'm seventeen, nearly eighteen. So really, I am leaving care, so.' When asked how she envisages this will go and when it will happen, Claire answers: 'It is depending on my emotional health and how I feel and how ready I am to leave.'

This is an interesting response in light of the mixed support she is receiving; the fact that the after-care charity is currently also supporting her hints at the fact that, although Claire may face a difficult transition from child to adult mental health care, she may also benefit from the 'staying put arrangement' – the entitlement to support until she is 25 years old (DfE, 2015). The above is interesting in light of what the after-care worker says in relation to the mental health and wellbeing of the young people she supports:

> With mental health and young people I would say … how would I define it? Let me think. I would say that the young people that we deal with don't have, not always but – their self-esteem is quite low, they're very … I find that they are quite reliant on the social workers, not in – emotionally but they get reliant on the fact that,

they can turn to someone – which is a good thing, obviously we know that but sometimes I think that they can shy away from doing something themselves, so like, the purpose of X [life-skills project] is to support them to do it themselves. I think sometimes that their mental health can stop them because they have got low self-esteem, they are not confident with certain aspects of their life, like maybe phoning someone for advice or sticking to appointments can sometimes be a challenge. And not realising actually, that every action has a consequence, I know that's quite hard to take, but actually, I know you are still a care leaver but you've still got to stick to some kind of rule, d'you know what I mean? For example, if you don't go the doctors you don't get seen. I know that seems harsh. But I think because they have constantly had a social worker, not running after them but looking out for them. Sometimes that ownership of their own life is removed from them. I'd say I'm quite, not harsh but I try to push them into doing it for themselves rather than me do it for them, which can sometimes be quite difficult for them to understand but you do get there eventually.

Thus, again help and support are discussed in terms of encouraging self-help and changing behaviour (Sohasky, 2015; Skinner & Thomas, 2018; Turner et al., 2015). Moreover, in line with the deserving/undeserving paradigm, self-responsibility is discussed in terms of 'you've got to stick to some kind of rule', ultimately leading to 'ownership of their own life'. As such, it could be argued that the notion of deservedness has fed into the creation of the welfare state, whose designers wanted it to be an insurance-based system, with a clear relationship between paying your dues and deserving help.

4.7 Sandy: aggressive, horrible, 'top dog' and confidence

Sandy is 18 years old and has a son who is nearly two. Sandy lives in supported accommodation with her son and is studying at college for a degree in social care. She suffers from stress-related anxiety and also refers to how she used to be 'aggressive' and 'horrible'. Sandy became a looked after child when she was 14 and was supported by the Young Person's Team, where she was allocated a social worker whom she worked well with. However after three years she was allocated a new social worker, and Sandy indicates that she cannot speak to this person and doesn't get along with her: 'Obviously, I do have a social worker, but I feel that I can't speak to her, as I don't get along with her at all.'

Sandy indicates that, as well as needing 'stress relief' and for someone to tell her to 'pick up your bum', she also needs to learn how to be polite and speak to people:

> as I used to be quite aggressive and horrible and stuff like that, and need to learn how to be more assertive and stuff like that. To speak properly and not get wound up and say things in the right way.

Thus, Sandy holds herself accountable, not only by referring to her laziness ('pick up your bum') but also by referring to her behaviour as someone who is 'quite aggressive and horrible'. By centralising 'saying things in the right way' she takes ownership of the fact that help and support are things that she has to earn, by learning to speak and behave properly, thus placing herself at the bottom of the 'deserving spectrum'. This approach also ignores the potential link between the stress she experiences, her mental health issues and 'bad' behaviours (Fong et al., 2018). Moreover, Sandy also appears to be held accountable and disadvantaged because of being a teenage mum – hinting at age, socio-economic and ethnic inequality in welfare provision (Jørgensen & Thomsen, 2018; Shah & Cook, 2008). This is illustrated by the following:

> So I wouldn't get paid because I was in college. Because I have a baby. You are not meant to have babies and go to college. So I was just. I went back to college and my money got stopped. But they turn around and say 'oh no, no, we will pay you then' cause obviously you get money for being a lone parent or being at college, but not both – so I sat there and went 'no'.

Here is what the after-care worker linked to the children's charity that is supporting Sandy has to say in relation to behaviour and mental health and wellbeing of care leavers:

> It can vary greatly. Umm I think we get a lot young people who feel they've got a reputation to keep up, so we've had a couple, particularly young ladies actually where the part of their mental health is around, 'if I am not top dog I am going to look weak'. So they will kind of act up to it even if they don't want to any more. Erm and I suppose mental health wise there are strategies for how they can feel okay to be who they want to be not who they feel they should be. For some it is when they move into properties and they are away from sort of the care system if you like that they

can then start to – and I'm not sure they always want to, but thoughts and reflexions start to come in about the life experiences they've had. Erm maybe that lack of – sometimes it is about lack of confidence. Sometimes it's not and sometimes it is just how do you deal with some of the things they may have been through, and even if the move into the actual care system wasn't particularly traumatic, they may have moved through foster carers and children's homes numerous times. So there may be that feeling of loss constantly going through that feeling of moving on, erm, so there can be so many different things and for some it is just, much lower level. It's is much more around the emotional health and how just getting into relationships that are healthy relationships rather than unhealthy. What friends they choose to have erm how they deal with peer pressure erm just friendships, how do you go about making new friendships what do you give of yourself cause you know do you go in saying: I've come from this ... you know at what point does it come up? When do you trust? There might be a lot of trust issues going on umm, I think it is very individual. But I think what comes through with a lot of them is around just almost like a listening ear, just somebody consistent that is there who will say 'you can do it'.

This care worker makes a link between mental health, attitude and behaviour by referring to mental health as 'if I am not top dog I am going to look weak'. At the same time the ongoing trauma is acknowledged, for example in relation to the 'life experiences they've had' – thus highlighting that narratives of help and support for vulnerable care leavers ('victims') are influenced by multiple strands, from self-responsibility on the one hand to centralising the needs of the vulnerable child on the other. This highlights that the complexity of definitions, conceptualisations and understandings of childhood – where some focus on the 'innocence of the child' and others view the child as an active agent in the perpetuation of pauperism through truancy and 'bad' behaviour – means that there is no neat fit between childhood and the deserving/undeserving paradigm (Morton, 2014).

4.8 Paul: extremely complicated mental health issues

Paul is 21 years old and has been in the care system since he was three. He is supported by an after-care charity and is no longer in touch with his foster parents. Paul describes himself in terms of being a lazy and difficult person: 'I'm such a lazy person' and 'I can be quite difficult sometimes, you know.' In addition to this, he also dislikes change: 'I'm not a big person on change, never have been, which is strange considering the things that I've changed.' At the same time, he is very grateful for the support provided by the after-care charity: 'they've helped me in a way to at least be a person to talk to' and 'they are trying to give me a lot of positives'. It is clear that this is very significant for Paul because 'I've never had anyone to talk to, like, I don't have any friends or anything like that, but I sort, don't really speak to anyone.' He describes his mental health as complicated: 'My mental health is extremely complicated, erm you known it's gone on for an extremely long time, but it's only sort of, in the last two years that it's come out'; 'I sort of have panic attacks and that kind of stuff.'

Thus, it could be argued that Paul's personal history of being in the care system with complex (mental health) needs – as well as care experiences that are marked by instability, disruption, loneliness and isolation – places him on the margins of society, with few privileges (see also Hood, 2016; Stein, 2006). This is also reflected in his narrative and those of the professionals who work with him. The following is an extract from an interview with an after-care worker:

> I'd say, I don't like to say it but some young people need quite a lot of support in that, around mental health and I think a lot of them find it quite hard to open up about things once you've built that trust in a relationship that normally comes with time I'd say. Once you start talking about things maybe in the past which they've been through which at the beginning they don't wanna talk about … Um, I think getting them to access the support that is available to them can be quite hard because they go through or they've been through counselling or different types of counselling before and they think that it hasn't worked for them and they don't want to try it again yet. As you get older things change in your life and different types, there is different types of resilience counselling and stuff out there for them it's just to make sure they know where it is and how to access it.
>
> […]
>
> I think some of our clients can become quite isolated I think in terms of if they're on benefits and they've been on benefits for a long time something like ESA [Employment and Support Allowance] for a disability or a mental health problem. Then it can be quite hard getting them to go out and seek things so we try to encourage them into things that will improve their confidence and self-esteem such as volunteering or getting them into maybe a part

time job and into education. That is quite a big thing for us that to make sure they're in something. Cause I do think that helps that, if you're sat at home and you haven't got a purpose or a routine it can be quite hard then to do anything.

Again, as well as discussing the needs of care leavers and related entitlement to support, there is also a clear sense of the fact that they have to earn this and that they have to be proactive, thus creating stratifications of support entitlement (Jørgensen & Thomsen, 2018).This focus on individual accountability and responsibility strongly resembles the deserving/undeserving criteria introduced by the 1834 Poor Law.

4.9 Conclusion

The data presented in this chapter highlights that in the care (or lack thereof) that some of the young people (e.g. Aaron and Katie) receive there is a sense of 'passing the buck' (see also Steffel et al., 2016). This is supported by research which suggests that in multi-agency contexts there is a tendency to pass the buck when there is a perceived risk of being accountable and/or possibly blamed for a bad outcome (see e.g. Morrison, 2016; Steffel et al., 2016). As with the previous chapter, by linking this to behaviour (e.g. being 'physically and verbally violent') and lack of resilience (e.g. being too reliant on social workers), the focus here is on a reductionist or isolated notion of the individual, rather than larger-scale social structures (e.g. issues around care and provision) (Dagnan, 2007; Toms, 2012). For example, in John's case, his bad behaviour takes centre stage, rather than the fact that supported accommodation is not yet forthcoming for him. Moreover, this narrative is also adopted by John himself when he focuses on his individual flaws, emotions and behaviour, rather than the dynamics in the immediate social context. Thus, both the historic case files in the previous chapter and the contemporary data presented here highlight a tendency to locate 'problems' (emotional and behavioural issues) in the individual, who is held accountable (Skinner & Thomas, 2018).

As such, the data presented in this chapter (as well as the previous one) evidences the ongoing influence of the deserving/undeserving paradigm in more than one way: for example, by locating problems not only in the individual but also in relation to the supported housing scheme, which is only available to those who have been in employment or education. This shows how the notion of deservedness has fed into the creation of the welfare state as an insurance-based system, with a clear relationship between paying your dues and deserving help (see also Shah & Cook, 2008). Moreover, by constructing young people as 'criminal children' and 'the naughtiest children in the city', the child is held accountable and positioned as beyond help (i.e. undeserving), This highlights inequalities in social care and NHS provision, creating new stratifications of exclusion and inclusion (Jørgensen & Thomsen, 2018; Shah & Cook, 2008). It could be argued that this goes hand in hand with a renewed focus on individual accountability and responsibility, which strongly resembles the deserving/undeserving criteria introduced by the Poor Law of 1834.

The data presented here also shines a light on the complexities around transitioning from child and adolescent mental health services (CAMHS) to adult mental health services (AMHS), leaving young people with mental health problems without professional support or a referral to an adult service (Hood, 2016; Sims-Schouten & Hayden, 2017; Winter, 2014). Research from the UK and the US shows that use of mental health services declines drastically when young people reach the age of 18 (over 60 per cent in the UK) (Paul et al., 2015). Thus, again help and support are discussed in terms of encouraging self-help and changing behaviour (Sohasky, 2015; Skinner & Thomas, 2018; Turner et al., 2015). Yet, as with the previous chapter, it should be noted that there is also evidence of care and support for the 'victims' presented in this chapter. For example, this is evident from the way in which ongoing trauma is acknowledged, in relation to 'life experiences they've had' – thus highlighting that narratives of help and support for vulnerable care leavers ('victims') are influenced by multiple strands, from self-responsibility on the one hand to centralising the needs of the vulnerable child on the other. Nevertheless, what the historic data from Chapter 3 and the contemporary data from this chapter also highlights is that similar narratives, constructs and realities around 'problematic children' and 'deservedness' when it comes to safeguarding and mental health support are as vivid today as they were in the late 1800s.

Note

1 Note that John neither attended nor was expelled from this school.

References

Action for Children, NCB and Children's Society (2017). *Turning the Tide: Reversing the Move to Late Intervention Spending in Children and Young People's Services.* https://www.childrenssociety.org.uk/sites/default/files/turning-the-tide.pdf.

Action for Children, NCB, Children's Society, NSPCC and Barnardo's (2018). *Children and Young People's Services, Funding and Spending 2010/2011 to 2017/2018.* https://www.childrenssociety.org.uk/sites/default/files/childrens-services-funding-csfa-briefing_final.pdf.

Akister, J., Owens, M. and Goodyer, I. (2010). Leaving care and mental health: outcomes for children in out-of-home care during the transition to adulthood. *Health Research Policy and Systems,* 8, art. 10. doi:10.1186/1478-4505-8-10.

Atherton, M. (2011). Deserving of charity or deserving of better? The continuing legacy of the 1834 Poor Law Amendment Act for Britain's deaf population. *Review of Disability Studies,* 7(3–4), 18–25.

Coman, W. and Devaney, J. (2011). Reflecting on outcomes for looked-after children: an ecological perspective. *Child Care in Practice,* 17(1), 37–53. doi:10.1080/13575279.2010.522976.

Community Care (2001). The Children Leaving Care Act explained. *Community Care,* 1. http://www.communitycare.co.uk/2001/09/12/the-children-leaving-care-act-explained/.

Dagnan, D. (2007), Psychosocial intervention for people with learning disabilities. *Advances in Mental Health and Learning Disabilities,* 1(2), 3–7.

DfE (Department for Education) (2015). Children looked after in England (including adoption and care leavers) year ending 31 March 2015. Statistical First Release (SFR) 34/2015, 1 October. https://www.gov.uk/government/uploads/system/uploads/attachment_data/file/464756/SFR34_2015_Text.pdf.

Dixon J. (2008). Young people leaving care: health, well-being and outcomes. *Child & Family Social Work,* 13, 207–217.

Eronen, T. (2011). Three stories about mother: narratives by women who have lived in care. *Child & Family Social Work,* 17(2), 66–74.

Fong, H.-F., Alegria, M., Bair-Merritt, M.H. and Beardslee, W. (2018). Factors associated with mental health services referrals for children investigated by child welfare. *Child Abuse & Neglect,* 79, 401–412. doi:10.1016/j.chiabu.2018.01.020.

Frost, N., Robinson, M. and Anning, A. (2005). Social workers in multi-disciplinary teams: issues and dilemmas for professional practice. *Child & Family Social Work,* 10(3), 187–196.

Hardwick, L. (2005), Fostering children with sexualised behaviour. *Adoption & Fostering,* 29(2), 33–43.

Holland, S. (2000). The assessment relationship: interactions between social workers and parents in child protection assessments. *British Journal of Social Work,* 30(2), 149–163.

Hood, R. (2016). How professionals talk about complex cases: a critical discourse analysis. *Child & Family Social Work,* 21(2), 125–135. doi:10.1111? cfs.12122.

Jørgensen, M.B. and Thomsen, T.L. (2018). 'Needed but undeserving': contestations of entitlement in the Danish policy framework on migration and integration. In: Fossum, J., Kastoryano, R. and Siim, B. (Eds.), *Diversity* and *Contestations over Nationalism in Europe and Canada.* London: Palgrave Macmillan, 337–364.

King, S.A. (2019). *Writing the Lives of the English Poor, 1750s–1830s.* Montreal: McGill-Queen's University Press.

Lindsay, M. (2014). *New Belongings: A Better Deal for Care Leavers. An Independent Evaluation of the New Belongings Project.* Bala: Care Leavers' Foundation. https://secure.toolkitfiles.co.uk/clients/23786/sitedata/files/Independent %20Ev.pdf.

Morrison, J. (2016). *Familiar Strangers, Juvenile Panics and the British Press: The Decline of Social Trust.* London: Palgrave Macmillan.

Morton, S. (2014). *Wisdom, Justice, Charity. Canadian Social Welfare through the Life of Jane B. Wisdom 1884–1975.* Toronto: University of Toronto Press.

NSPCC (2016). *Children in care: emotional wellbeing and mental health.* https://www.nspcc.org.uk/preventing-abuse/child-protection-system/children-in-care/emotional-wellbeing-of-children-in-care/.

Paul, M., Street, C., Wheeler, N. and Singh, S.P. (2015). Transition to adult services for young people with mental health needs: a systematic review. *Clinical Child Psychology and Psychiatry*, 20(3), 436–457.

Priest, P., Dunn, C., Hackett, J. and Wills, K. (2011). How can mental health professionals best be supported in working with people who experience significant stress? *Journal of Mental Health*, 20(6), 543–554.

Rey, J.M., Assumpção, F.B., Bernad, C.A., Çuhadaroğlu, F.C., Evans, B., Fung, D., Harper, G., Loidreau, L., Ono, Y., Pūras, D., Remschmidt, H., Robertson, B., Rusakoskaya, O.A. and Schleimer, K. (2015). History of child and adolescent psychiatry. In: Rey, J.M. (Ed.), *IACAPAP e-Textbook of Child and Adolescent Mental Health.* Geneva: International Association for Child and Adolescent Psychiatry and Allied Professions, 1–67.

Richardson, J. and Lelliott, P. (2003). Mental health of looked after children. *Advances in Psychiatric Treatment*, 9(4), 249–257.

Shah, S.M. and Cook, D.G. (2008). Socio-economic determinants of casualty and NHS Direct use. *Journal of Public Health*, 30(1), 75–81.

Sims-Schouten, W. and Hayden, C. (2017). Mental health and wellbeing of care leavers: making sense of their perspectives. *Child & Family Social Work*, 24(4), 1480–1487.

Sims-Schouten, W. and Riley, S. (2018). Presenting critical realist discourse analysis as a tool for making sense of service users' accounts of their mental health problems. *Qualitative Health Research*, 29(7). doi:10.1177/1049732318818824.

Singh, S.P. and Tuomainen, H. (2015). Transition from child to adult mental health services: needs, barriers, experiences and new models of care. *World Psychiatry*, 14(3), 358–361. doi:10.1002/wps.20266.

Skinner, A. and Thomas, N. (2018). 'A pest to society': the Charity Organisation Society's domiciliary assessments into the circumstances of poor families and children. *Children & Society*, 32, 133–144. doi:10.1111/chso.12237.

Sohasky, K.E. (2015). Safeguarding the interests of the state from defective delinquent girls. *Journal of the History of Behavioral Sciences, 52(*1), 20–40. doi:10.1002/jhbs.21765.

Steffel, M., William, E.F. and Perrmann-Graham, J. (2016). Passing the buck: delegating choices to others to avoid responsibility and blame. *Organizational Behavior and Human Decision Processes*, 135, 32–44.

Stein, M. (2006). Research review: young people leaving care. *Child and Family Social Work*, 11(3), 273–279.

Stein, M. (2008). Resilience and young people leaving care. *Child Care in Practice*, 14(1), 35–44.

Stein, M. and Carey, K. (1986). *Leaving Care*. Oxford: Blackwell.

Stein, M. and Dumaret, A.-C. (2011). The mental health of young people aging out of care and entering adulthood: exploring the evidence from England and France. *Children and Youth Services Review*, 33(12), 2504–2511.

Toms, J. (2012). Political dimensions of 'the psychosocial': the 1948 International Congress on Mental Health and the mental hygiene movement. *History of the Human Sciences*, 25(5), 91–106.

Turner, J., Hayward, R., Angel, K., Fulford, B., Hall, J., Millard, C. and Thomson, M. (2015). The history of mental health services in modern England: practitioner memories and the direction of future research. *Medical History*, 59(4), 599–624. doi:10.1017/mdh.2015.48.

Ungar, M. (2002). *Playing at Being Bad: The Hidden Resilience of Troubled Teens*. Halifax, NS: Pottersfield Press.

Ungar, M. (2004). *Nurturing Hidden Resilience in Troubled Youth*. Toronto: University of Toronto Press.

Ungar, M. (2005). *A Handbook for Working with Children and Youth: Pathways to Resilience across Cultures and Contexts*. Thousand Oaks, CA: Sage.

Waechter, R., Kumanayaka, D. and Angus-Yamada, C. (2019). Maltreatment history, trauma symptoms and research reactivity among adolescents in child protection services. *Child and Adolescent Psychiatry and MentalHealth*, 13(13). doi.org/10.1186/s13034-019-0270-7.

WHO (2012). Risks to mental health: an overview of vulnerabilities and risk factors. Background paper by WHO Secretariat for the development of a comprehensive mental health action plan. http://www.who.int/mental_health/mhgap/risks_to_mental_health_EN_27_08_12.pdf.

Winter, K. (2014). Understanding and supporting young children's transitions into state care: Schlossberg's transition framework and child-centred practice. *British Journal of Social Work*, 44(2), 401–417.

Zehr, H. (2015). *The Little Book of Restorative Justice*. New York: Good Books.

5 Good practice and bad practice
Lessons learnt

Although child safeguarding practices have developed enormously since Victorian times, and awareness of mental health problems and disorders in childhood has risen, the proportion of those who need mental health and social care but who do not receive support that meets their needs remains high (Cylus et al., 2018; Memon et al., 2016). This so-called 'treatment gap' has resulted in substantial disparities in access to mental health services for what the World Health Organization (WHO) refers to as 'vulnerable groups', such as children growing up in care and young care leavers (Van Keer et al., 2017; Sims-Schouten et al., 2019; Waechter et al., 2019; Zarse et al., 2019). Here, the term 'vulnerable groups' is used to refer to individuals/groups who are made vulnerable by the situations and environments they are exposed to, rather than through any inherent weakness or lack of capacity.

In this chapter, I will reflect on current and past practices with a focus on safeguarding and mental health support in childhood. Drawing on the data presented in Chapters 3 and 4 and wider debates in this area, I will provide insights into the legacy of the deserving/undeserving paradigm, specifically in relation to the most vulnerable children with the most complex (mental health) needs and damaging pre-care (care and post-care) experiences, referred to as 'victims' by Mike Stein (2006). Moreover, I will take a closer look at the theme and construct of 'beyond help' in relation to these children, as well as providing insights into multi-agency support, practices and failures in support services here.

Following this, I will shed light on the meaning of childhood, reflecting on historic and contemporary narratives around childhood. As well as considering historic and contemporary safeguarding practices and mental health support for vulnerable children, there is also need to look into how this can affect subsequent generations through intergenerational and transgenerational trauma, which will be discussed further in the final section. Ultimately, this chapter aims to provide examples of good and bad practices with vulnerable children and families, with a view to finding and identifying ways forward.

5.1 The legacy of the deserving/undeserving paradigm in practice with vulnerable children

When it comes to the situations and environments that children in care and young care leavers are exposed to, both now and in late Victorian times, it is not only deprivation, neglect and abuse that matter, but also perceptions of 'deservedness' (in relation to receiving help and support). The latter is important as evidence suggests that, in light of ongoing cuts to budgets and resources, as well as stigma, decisions tend to be made about who can be helped and who can't (Atherton, 2011; Jørgensen & Thomson, 2018; Sims-Schouten et al., 2019. Current procedures regarding child safeguarding often dismiss historical and structural mechanisms in unequal practices, locating problems in families and parenting instead. Practitioner perceptions and decisions around who should get help or is deserving of support also need to be considered here. For example, Holland (2000) found that clients (usually mothers) were seen as deserving of help and motivated to change if they agreed with the social worker, whereas clients who didn't agreed with the social worker were construed as 'risky'. In light of ongoing cuts to services, this may also mean that some families miss out due to not 'fitting the profile' or having complex needs that are hard to cater to. As a result 'complex' families/children are sent from pillar to post. As can be seen from the data presented in this book, the dominant narrative adopted by agencies and social services often appears to be one that stresses that 'this is out of my remit' and 'not my job'. This practice and tendency to pass the buck, in multi-agency contexts, can often be seen to be happening when there is a perceived risk of being held accountable and/or possibly blamed for a bad outcome (Morrison, 2016; Steffel et al., 2016).

Rather than reflecting on where practice may have gone wrong, leading to vulnerable children missing out on the support they so desperately need, the debate more often than not revolves around (bad) parenting, neglect or abuse as causal factors. Within this, early intervention and prevention are promoted as the 'holy grail', as something that can cure and remedy bad parenting practices and related early childhood experiences. Here the main focus is on the practice of early intervention/prevention itself, with less emphasis on reflections on practice and/or potential stigma inherent in this (Choudbury & Moses, 2016; Cowan et al., 2016). Additionally, the focus on early intervention/prevention sets child safeguarding aside from more 'heavy-end' child protection, or tertiary and 'quaternary' prevention as Munro (2011) terms it (see also Whittaker & Havard, 2015).

It should however be noted that, in light of austerity and cuts to funding, it is not only vulnerable children and families who suffer. Despite examples of failure in practice (e.g. the cases of Baby P and Victoria Climbié), for most safeguarding practitioners/professionals a professional ethic of helping and supporting service users is at the forefront of their practice. Yet practice is negatively affected by ongoing cuts to (referral) services, the rising nature of thresholds, staff shortages and lack of time to spend with families (Höjer et al., 2017; Frost et al., 2017). Thus, there is a need to reflect on larger structural mechanisms and causal factors – political, institutional and social-cultural – that impact practice and related perceptions regarding 'deserving' and 'undeserving' children and families.

As a society, we create situations and environments for practice with vulnerable children; these practices evolve, slowly, but can also be ambivalent and contradictory (Lyndon, 2019; Sims-Schouten et al., 2019). For example, whilst we recognise and respond to sexual abuse, treating this as a child protection and safeguarding issue, there are also cases – such as the sexual exploitation cases in Rotherham and other cities in the UK – where the victims are blamed and too little is done too late (Delap, 2015; Ellis, 2020; Morrison, 2016). Thus, practice evolves slowly and with ambivalence, suffers reversals of fortune and varies widely (Whittaker & Havard, 2015). Perceptions and different portrayals of 'imperfect' children and families, in terms of their mental health, morality and behaviour, also play a role in the way in which 'problem children' and 'problem families' have been constructed over the ages (Sims-Schouten et al., 2019; Wynter, 2015). Moreover, here a link is made between 'imperfect', 'problematic' and 'undeserving', thereby justifying why certain families and children don't get support.

These perceptions are underpinned by strong and powerful discursive labels that support the case that some people are simply incorrigible, ignoring the role of structural mechanisms and inequalities, as discussed in Chapter 2 (Cowan et al., 2016; Houston, 2010; Sales, 2002; Sims-Schouten & Riley, 2014). Take for example Rebecca Wynter's (2015) analysis of perceptions and approaches towards mental deficiency in the Monyhull Colony, a mental hospital in Birmingham (West Midlands) that originated in 1904. Wynter discusses the case of the B. family: the mother is described and construed as having 'repeated attacks of insanity' and her children as 'mentally defective', with one an 'epileptic imbecile' and another as having 'fits of uncontrollable passion, and will probably become insane'; meanwhile the father is a criminal and in prison. As Wynter argues, and as can be seen from the data presented in Chapter 3 of this book, a welter of characteristics are applied to mental deficiency here, such as 'immoral', 'imbecile', 'hysterical'. Moreover, both in the historical data and the contemporary data in Chapters 3 and 4, a catalogue of characteristics are used to describe 'problematic children'. For example, in Chapter 3 there is talk of a child who 'turned out very bad', and reference is made to a child having a 'mental deficiency', 'immoral tendencies and 'unsatisfactory characteristics' or being an 'imbecile'. In Chapter 4 reference is made to 'criminal children' and wanting to be 'top dog', as well as being 'quite reliant on social workers'. Thus, in both the historic and contemporary datasets there are examples of situations where it seems the child is blamed for what can be perceived as the consequences of trauma, abuse and neglect. This will be discussed further in the next section.

5.2 Beyond help and beyond hope: problematic children

The conflicting narrative between child safeguarding/protection and deservedness in Britain has been profoundly shaped by recurrent episodes of moral panic and media scandalmongering, usually centring on individual cases and examples (Whittaker & Havard, 2015; Morrison, 2016; Sims-Schouten et al., 2019). For example, consider documentaries, such as *Saints and Scroungers*, broadcast on BBC 1, and Channel 5's *On Benefits and Proud*, which almost always focus on burdensome and large problem families. Some of this can also be seen in earlier cases: in Chapter 3, for example, Harry is described as 'an extremely lazy boy'; and in Chapter 4 Paul describes himself as 'lazy person' who can be 'quite difficult sometimes', rendering both boys as less deserving of help and support.

The construct 'deservedness' is tricky in light of the current focus on prevention/early intervention in practice with children and families, as it means that some may be perceived as 'problematic' and 'beyond help' from the word go. Comparison between the two datasets presented in Chapters 3 and 4 highlights that children with mental health issues are especially construed as 'problematic', both by practitioners (56 per cent of the adults in the historic correspondence and 46 per cent of the practitioners interviewed in the contemporary dataset) and the children themselves (11 per cent for dataset 1 and 42 per cent for dataset 2).

In both datasets links can be found between the stigmas and bias surrounding the participants and their non-discursive realities. For example, there is evidence that the children in both studies were on the margins of society, with little help and support available. This lack of support was justified through constructions of them being 'problematic children' with 'complex' needs and 'beyond hope'. Yet these children are also 'victims' and 'vulnerable', not because of an inherent weakness but because of the situations they find themselves in (Hood, 2016; Sims-Schouten et al., 2019). Moreover, in line with Ungar (2002, 2004, 2005), it could be argued that their 'delinquent' and 'disordered' behaviour could signify hidden pathways to resilience through the only means available to them. Nevertheless, in both datasets there is a strong sense that how children act out their trauma and associated behaviour becomes the problem, rather than the trauma itself and what caused it (Burchell, 2019; Hood, 2016; Sims-Schouten et al., 2019).

Children and young people may be reluctant to disclose and share information, and their behaviours that are a response to abuse, neglect and being in a risky situation are often misunderstood as them acting out and misbehaving, rather than them being at risk (Waechter et al., 2019; Zarse et al., 2019). As such, their complex mental health issues and related behaviours are labelled as risky, rather than as a consequence of being at risk. Yet, something that is presented as problematic because of the complex and varied symptoms and behaviours often has as part of the pattern underlying histories of abuse, neglect and trauma, which are often not recognised (Baldwin et al., 2019; Waechter et al., 2019).

This approach to labelling and blaming the child is not unique to care-experienced children and young people. For example, when it comes to refugees and asylum seekers, there is evidence that their ethnic background and migration status affect their perceived deservedness (Kootstra, 2016). Moreover, for child refugees there is the added element of being expected to be 'genuine' children, and truly deserving of help and support. For example, whilst there is evidence that pictures of vulnerable and dying child refugees evoke feelings of compassion, there is also a sense of hostility towards child refugees who may not be 'genuine', either due to their perceived age (too old to be a child) or behaviour (Ala, 2018; Kushner & Knox, 2012). A number of child refugees entered the UK following the Dubs Amendment to the UK's Immigration Act of 2016 (named after Labour peer Lord Alfred Dubs), and this was widely documented in the news (McLaughlin, 2018). Yet, at the same time, the campaign highlighted an element of scrutiny and suspicion of 'unchildlike children' and the criminalisation of undocumented migrants.

Popular discourse around deservedness, e.g. in relation to the vulnerability and/or malevolence of different types of children and their families, often acts as a locus for manifestations of stigma, prejudices and deeper-seated anxiety – including perceptions of lifestyle choices, socio-economic background and cultural characteristics (Morrison, 2016), both now and in the past. The dominant overarching image of vulnerable child refugees does not allow any room for a more nuanced understanding of the experiences of individual children, such as behaviours resulting from the trauma of being separated from their families or abused in their new homes (Kushner & Knox, 2012; Morgan, 2020). As such, the taken-for-granted and expected innocence, vulnerability and gratitude of these children is central to the overarching discourse, and fails to consider the muddled category of childhood, youth or adolescence (McLaughlin, 2018; Sims-Schouten et al., 2019). In this way, the construct of the 'unchildlike' asylum-seeking child can be seen as a further instance of what Elizabeth Brown (2011, 362) calls the 'fracturing of childhood'. Here, the concept 'child refugee/asylum seeker' is synonymous with the stereotype of juvenile delinquency, and placed within a 'classed/racialised hierarchy' that stigmatises these young people as less important than other children (McLaughlin, 2018; Hopkins & Hill, 2010).

Again, as with the data presented in this book, comparisons can be made between past and contemporary practices, in this case in relation to child migration schemes (Constantine, 2013; Lynch, 2015). For example, judgements fuelled by the deserving/undeserving paradigm and eugenics coloured decisions regarding which children should be sent to Canada as part of the Canadian British Home Child movement (1869–1932) and to Australia as part of the Australian Child Migration scheme (1940–1970). Some of this could be traced back to the focus on heredity, environment and moral purity of the time (Hall, 1904; Lynch, 2019). The Waifs and Strays Society, discussed in Chapter 3, was one of the philanthropic organisations involved in child migration schemes, and sent approximately 3500 children to Canada between 1883 and 1937 (House of Commons, 2018; Higginbotham, 2017; Lynch, 2015). The Waifs and Strays Society emigration archives held at the Library and Archives Canada (LAC) in Ottawa refer to 'hereditary pauperism' in relation to the Australian and USA boarding-out schemes. Moreover, a letter from one of the receiving homes in Canada refers to 'a troublesome girl [being] pushed through' – here the 'trouble' appears to be related to bed-wetting. Moreover, children are described in relation to 'behaviour', 'deficiency' and 'work-ethic'.

Similar constructs can be seen in relation to the *Kindertransport* programme, the rescue effort that took place between 1938 and 1940 to take thousands of Jewish children to safety ahead of World War Two. There is evidence that here, again, the (Jewish) migrant child was often seen as synonymous with 'less worthy' (Grenville, 2012; Kushner & Knox, 2012; McDonald, 2018). For example, Grenville (2012, 4) highlights how the British authorities treated the Jewish child refugees as temporary immigrants, driven by demographic considerations and the reluctance to 'replenish that good white stock with Jewish racial material'. Moreover, Kushner and Knox argue that the image of the *Kindertransport* that has survived in British public memory (i.e. the notion that the Jewish child refugees were welcomed) is selective and flawed, and instead the programme was marked by marginalisation, refused entry and exclusion (see also McDonald, 2018). The next section will take a closer look at the complex and dynamic matrix inherent in multi-agency and multidisciplinary approaches, with a focus on inclusive (and exclusive) practice.

5.3 'Not my job' and multidisciplinary approaches that work

Over the decades there have been a number of safeguarding and mental health reforms, often in answer to major problematic events – such as the tragic and horrific death of Victoria Climbié at the hands of her aunt and boyfriend in 2000, leading to the Laming report in 2003 (see also Balen & Masson, 2007). Some of the safeguarding reforms have been critiqued for increasing state surveillance in the lives of children and young people whilst at the same time achieving little to secure adequate protection for children and young people at highest risk of significant harm (see for example Munro, 2011; Thane, 2012; Tisdall, 2017). The focus on early intervention and prevention, while praiseworthy in intentions, in reality is underpinned by the risky assumption that professionals can accurately predict which children will be problematic (Balen & Masson, 2007; Cowan et al., 2016; Slack & Webber, 2008). Moreover, the assumption here is that practitioners and professionals are in a position to intervene effectively, using coercion if necessary, and change the course of children's development, and that there will be adequate resources to meet the needs identified through screening (Munro, 2007, 53).

Similarly, while there are a number of trauma-assessment/screening tools for children/young people – such as the Child and Adolescent Needs and Strengths (CANS), the Child PTSD [Post-Traumatic Stress Disorder] Symptom Scale (CPSS) or the Childhood Trauma

Questionnaire(CTQ) – these often include standardised (clinical) interviews, measures and behavioural observations/assessments, with the potential to lead to the exclusion of children/young people who don't fit the picture, such as those with complex problems (de Roos et al., 2011; Waechter et al., 2019; Zarse et al., 2019). For those young people who receive services, needs-led treatment is not the norm, and many adolescent interventions are either downward extensions of adult programmes or upward extensions of child programmes (Akister et al., 2010; Fong et al., 2018; Sims-Schouten & Hayden, 2017).

Research on adverse childhood experiences and trauma has highlighted that all care-experienced children will have experienced trauma in some form (Jones et al., 2018). For example, roughly 69 per cent of children in care have experienced neglect, 48 per cent physical abuse, 37 per cent emotional abuse and 23 per cent sexual abuse (Chambers, 2017; Zarse et al., 2019); yet there is limited research around children/ young people's perceptions of trauma and their related needs. My previous research (Sims-Schouten & Edwards, 2016; Sims-Schouten & Hayden, 2017) highlights the value of engaging with (young) people in understanding their needs and developing systems of formal/informal support. Yet, despite calls for greater involvement of young people in services that affect them, in reality this is often tokenistic or a 'tick box' exercise (Tisdall, 2017; Woodcock Ross, 2016). Thus, there is a need to centralise the needs and voices of children and young people. Moreover, judging the complex behaviour and mental health issues of the child, rather than the child's background and early experiences, appears to be a feature of state agencies and is something that needs to be picked up with professionals and managers working in mental health and social care (Hood, 2014, 2016; Munro, 2011). This also includes the acknowledgement that those 'badly behaved' children and young people deserve our understanding and support (Baldwin et al., 2019; Waechter et al., 2019). The same applies to children and young people as asylum seekers, who are often treated as immigration offenders first and traumatised children second (Hopkins & Hill, 2010).

Here, the lack of funds and resources, as discussed earlier, may have two specific consequences. First, it may push the focus more towards interventions with a focus on self-management, such as mindfulness practice, which can also be described as an 'inward-focused goal-oriented practice concerned with individualised and neoliberalist self-improvement of children and adolescents' (Choudbury & Moses, 2016, 592). Here 'individual-oriented practice' becomes the dominant intervention over alternative solutions for young people within welfare and education policy. Having said this, when applied properly and sensitively, mindfulness in education can assist children and young people in developing relationships and critically examining their circumstances, which could ultimately aid their mental health and wellbeing (Choudbury et al., 2015; Sharf, 2014).

Second, in light of budget cuts and a cap on resources, social services may prioritise provision to younger children because they consider older children to be more resilient and more able to cope with the effects of abuse (Action for Children et al., 2018). Yet, here the inherent danger is that neglect of this age group will be overlooked. Moreover, practitioners may assume that children are making choices relevant to their chronological age, when in fact it should be acknowledged that children who have experienced trauma, neglect and abuse tend to function at a younger emotional or developmental age (Cowie, 2019; Zarse et al., 2019). This means that there may be more of a tendency to judge older children's 'bad' behaviour, as can be seen from the data in Chapters 3 and 4, leading to exclusion from practices/support. For example, what might seem to be 'bad' behaviour among older children – such as 'being top dog', 'kicking off', truanting and self-harm – may mask underlying problems and be a symptom that a child is at risk.

Rather than construing these young people as 'beyond help', the role of social care support workers, social workers and charities is to be a critical friend and challenge the initial judgements and dig beneath the presenting behaviour. Thus, there is a need for greater awareness of the fact that older children may also be vulnerable and 'in need', which includes the need to assess the needs of those children and offer support. Additionally, there is a need to reflect on the way in which separated unaccompanied children with insecure immigration status are treated, and eradicate the current beliefs and procedures that those children/young people cannot be cared for and supported until they have claimed (and been approved for) asylum (Ala, 2018; Carrillo, 2018; Sales, 2002). This also includes reflecting on government spending priorities as it is all too easy to point the finger at 'failing disciplines and practices', whilst there is a need to look at the larger picture.

What this chapter and the research in this book have shown is that the deserving/undeserving paradigm permeates historical and contemporary practices, leading certain children and families to consistently miss out on support. Here it is important to focus upon key perceptions and conceptions of childhood because, as Prout (2019, 314) argues, 'In the timescale of historical change childhood often emerges as a crucial component of key social issues.' This includes drawing attention to wellbeing and inclusive practice in childhood, and centralising the voice of the child. It follows that there is a need for a reflection on and re-engagement with childhood as something that is authentic and unique to children, centralising notions such as 'child-centeredness', 'children's voices' and 'children's perspectives' (Spyrou, 2019; Stryker et al., 2019). In the next section I will reflect on the changing perceptions of childhood.

5.4 Rethinking childhood and youth

> The immaturity of children is a biological fact of life, but the ways in which this immaturity is understood and made meaningful is a fact of culture
>
> (Prout & James, 1997, 7)

In the preface to her book *Forgotten Children: Parent–Child Relations from 1500 to 1900* Linda Pollock (1983, viii) highlights that:

> The history of childhood is an area so full of errors, distortion and misinterpretation that I thought it vital, if progress were to be made, to supply a clear review of the information on childhood contained in such sources as diaries and autobiographies.

It is a commonly held belief that the concept of childhood did not emerge until the 18th and 19th centuries, that the 20th and 21st are 'centuries of the child' (Prout, 2019; Stryker et al., 2019); but the question is – are they? Below I will tackle this question by first looking at historic concepts of childhood, followed by a reflection on childhood in contemporary society. The (late) Victorian times, in which Chapter 3 of this book is set, are generally perceived as marking the emergence of the modern attitude to childhood – one in which the innocence of children is recognised and childhood is perceived as a separate phase to adulthood (Prout & James, 1997). This change coincides (to an extent) with the child rescue movement and the establishment of philanthropic institutions, such as Barnardo's and the Waifs and Strays Society, the passing of various children's rights Acts and the establishment of the NSPCC (Gingell, 2001; Hacking, 1991; Higginbotham, 2017; Melling et al. 1997; NSPCC, 2016). At the same time, Victorian times are often portrayed in terms of being 'harsh', especially for the poor, working-class child. It should however be noted that the image of the uncaring and emotionally distant Victorians does not necessarily reflect the ideology and practice of the time; and, as with current practices and ideologies, it is crucial to see this in light of different institutional, religious and philanthropic approaches, as discussed in Chapter 1 (Moss et al., 2017; Sims-Schouten et al., 2019).

Within contemporary society the needs of the child supposedly take central place in the policy and practices of welfare, medical and educational institutions. Yet, as mentioned earlier, any complacency about childhood and children's place in society is misplaced, as the very concept of childhood has become problematic during the last few decades (Stryker et al., 2019; Thomas, 2019). Some even argue that 'childhood is disappearing' (Hendrick, 1997; Spyrou, 2019). Debates about child abuse, child protection, safeguarding and mental health and wellbeing are now deeply embedded in discourses about childhood – what it is, what it means (Cradock, 2014; Stryker et al., 2019). Yet, the very notion of 'child abuse' implies an erosion of power and takes the nature of the child for granted, as this is premised on the notion of the 'child' yet negates the fact that this also reflects young (er), small(er) and weak(er) persons (Kitzinger, 1997). It follows that child safeguarding practices are to an extent underpinned by theories of pollution (Boyden, 1997; Thomas, 2019), i.e. the concept that adult society undermines childhood innocence, and therefore children must be protected from social dangers.

At the same time, there is no such notion as 'child mental health', and mental illness in childhood and related perceptions are still very much grounded in our understanding of and perceptions regarding 'adult mental health'(Rey et al., 2015). Thus, despite a growing awareness of the fact that children are going through various developmental stages, this is not necessarily reflected in understanding regarding 'child abuse' (suggesting that 'child' is a concept rather than a developmental phase consisting of different stages/ages) and 'mental health and wellbeing in childhood' (still often grounded in adult perceptions and terminology) (Cradock, 2014; Hacking, 1991; Kitzinger, 1997).

In addition to this, current perceptions and practices reflect historical attitudes towards social pathology, which is both punitive and judgemental in nature. This is reflected for example in views surrounding immoral behaviour in children, judgements about 'bad' behaviour of children and ignorance of the correlation between certain 'bad' behaviours and an abusive past (Atherton, 2011; Stryker et al., 2019). For example, a sexually abused child may bring to their foster placement challenging behaviours, some of which will be sexualised, and foster carers may inappropriately manage the situation by punishing the child for their 'immoral tendencies' (Fisher et al., 2000;

Hardwick, 2005). See also the example of 'impure talk' provided in Chapter 3. Moreover, as mentioned earlier, and as can be seen in Chapter 4, there is evidence that social workers view their clients as resistant and 'risky' if they disagree with them and/or lack motivation to change (Holland, 2000).

Links are also made to social and economic factors that contribute to the 'respectability' of families and children, such as in the case of the sexual exploitation scandals discussed earlier where girls as young as 13 were abused and described by professionals as 'out of control', 'streetwise' and 'akin to prostitutes' (Delap, 2015; Morrison, 2016). Another example is the suicide of a 14-year-old girl from Canada's First Nations community, described by professionals as 'street savvy' and, ignoring her distress, revealing a dysfunctional child protection system that is not reaching the children who need it most (Sims-Schouten et al., 2019; Turpel-Lafond, 2014). Thus the unwillingness and inability to distinguish between the 'poor child', 'the criminal child' and 'the insane child' remains; and it is here that the ongoing influence of the deserving/undeserving paradigm can be seen in our approach to vulnerable children, historically and today, as their lives often overlap(ped) in many ways (Hurren, 2015; King, 2019).

Social and welfare policy can be extremely exclusive, penalising and uncompromising in its application, especially when resources are scarce. It can have the effect of punishing or even criminalising the childhoods of the poor for the simple reason that families living in poverty may not be able to reach certain required/expected standards (Boyden, 1997; Lyndon, 2019). Thus, in a sense child welfare has evolved as a means by which one group in society imposes their values on others; as statutory welfare bodies are mainly run by the urban wealthy, it is they who are in charge of interpreting legislation (Cox, 2013; Cylus et al., 2018; Jehu et al., 2018). It is in this light that we need to see the ongoing trauma in families – passed on from generation to generation, often leading to complex issues, including re-referral to social services. As Baum (2012, 40) highlights: 'The body of a survivor marks trauma on the descendants in the simple fact of its being.' This will be discussed further in the next section.

5.5 Intergenerational/transgenerational trauma

When I was quite young, on a family picnic, we went swimming and I asked my father what happened to his feet. He simply said, 'A wagon wheel ran over my feet when I was working on a farm.' His feet troubled him all his life and were a daily reminder of his time in care. He tried to enlist in WWII in order to get to England but was refused because of his feet. Decades later, he confided that his feet were mangled because he had to wear women's boots while he was in foster care in England for 8 years. Many other British Home Children in care carried their physical scars as well as emotional in silence all their lives. Patterns of behaviour were inadvertently passed on to their children as inter-generational trauma. (Email correspondence from a descendant of a British Home Child, 10 December 2019)

I believe I was born into trauma – my mother's childhood trauma was passed down to her children – I felt out of place – with no roots and angry that my mother wouldn't talk about her past – it took her until she was well into her 70s before she started opening up. (Email correspondence with descendant of a British Home Child, 2 July 2019)

Pre-care experiences, as well as care and leaving care experiences, can be difficult and traumatic (Duncalf, 2010). Many young people, especially those referred to by Stein (2006) as 'victims', leave care unprepared, traumatised and with a wealth of problems, including difficulties with education/employment, mental health and homelessness (Dixon, 2008; Sims-Schouten & Hayden, 2017). Yet, there is little acknowledgement that some of these issues will have consequences across the life course. There is a need to develop knowledge and understanding of intergenerational and transgenerational trauma when it comes to children who grow up in the care system and displaced children. Whilst intergenerational trauma refers to the specific experience of trauma across familial generations, transgenerational trauma refers to shared group trauma (Pearrow & Cosgrove, 2009; George, 2015). Both are controversial terms, used to highlight that chronic and acute trauma can be long-lasting and can be transferred from one generation to another via complex post-traumatic stress disorder (PTSD) mechanisms.

So far the field of research around transgenerational trauma has predominantly focused on symptoms and treatment of concentration camp syndrome – in response to the observation that large numbers of children of Holocaust survivors were seeking treatment in psychiatric clinics (Baum, 2012; Fossion et al., 2003) – as well as post-traumatic slave syndrome, the passing on of psychological and emotional trauma from slavery (George, 2015; Leigh et al., 2017). Moreover, a number of studies have looked at intergenerational trauma in indigenous populations, e.g. in relation to residential schools in Canada, a network of boarding schools in the 1870s–1990s for indigenous people created for the purpose of cultural genocide by removing children from the influence of their own culture and assimilating them into the dominant Canadian culture (Bombay et al., 2014; George, 2015; Leigh et al., 2017). Students in the residential school system were faced with harsh discipline and abuse from teachers and administrators, including sexual and physical assault.

The research around intergenerational and transgenerational trauma can be located within medical and social models/frameworks. For example, whilst some studies have looked at epigenetic transmission – the notion that one's environment and external experiences can impact on cellular activity (e.g. Blake and Watson, 2016) – others have studied transmission during pregnancy (e.g. Kinsella & Monk, 2009), as well as psychological and social causes and consequences (Cowan et al., 2016).

Despite the controversy around intergenerational/transgenerational trauma theory, it is safe to assume that young people leaving the care system may experience long-lasting (mental health) problems (Waechter et al., 2019). Yet, there is little research that looks at care leavers' experiences beyond the age of 25. An exception is Duncalf (2010), although the focus of this work is not so much on intergenerational/transgenerational trauma, but more on viewing the care experience through the retrospective lens of care leavers up to the age of 78.

Care-experienced young people can suffer from acute and chronic trauma, as well as PTSD (Waechter et al., 2019; Zarse et al., 2019). Here it is important to reflect on definitions and conceptualisations: according to the fifth edition of the *Diagnostic and Statistical Manual of Mental Disorders* (DSM-5), PTSD falls under trauma and stressor related disorders, and includes exposure to a traumatic or stressful event as a diagnostic criterion (Dziegielewski, 2016). Yet, these symptoms fail to address more contextual, systemic, and structural issues, including how trauma is perceived and experienced by young people.

Edith Stein, a phenomenologist and philosopher, highlights how meaningful experiences can both transpire between people, and within persons. She describes the first as a 'mental phenomenon', referring to the 'sameness of meaning' requiring an interpersonal matrix, and the second as a 'sentient phenomenon', referring to sensations, sensibilities and emotions that require an intrapersonal matrix (Stein, 2000, xiii). Linking to this to the critical realist ontology discussed in Chapter 2 and applied to the data in Chapters 3 and 4 highlights a need to locate experiences of intergenerational/transgenerational trauma within the 'real' (exploring causal mechanisms of events), the 'empirical' (how events are experienced by individuals) and the 'actual' (events and processes that occur and are in place, such as formal and informal support systems) (Bhaskar, 1989, 2014).

Specifically, the dominant focus on intra-individual factors in trauma and mental health issues ignores the potential intergenerational impact of trauma. Other aspects need to be recognised here as well, such as the fact that caring for or being cared for by a traumatised person can lead to secondary traumatic stress (Slack & Webber, 2008). Although it is difficult to pinpoint specific factors that 'cause' inter-generational trauma, it is possible to identify mechanisms that play a role here. For example, Ancharoff et al. (1998) identified four possible mechanisms and causes associated with transgenerational trauma.

- First is 'silence', where the parent/care giver does not vocalise what they have been through, but the child nevertheless senses the parent/care giver's fragility and/or is taught to avoid topics or sti-muli that might upset the parent/care giver. As a consequence, the child's anxiety accelerates as she/he is unable to seek out help/comfort from the parent.
- Second is 'overdisclosure', where a parent/care giver overwhelms the child by explaining their trauma in graphic detail, leaving the child terrified.
- Third is 'identification', which happens when a child is con-tinuously exposed to the post-traumatic symptoms of their parent/care giver, and begins to identify with and imitate the symptoms in order to connect with the parent.
- Finally, there is 're-enactment', which prefers to the mechanism asso-ciated with transmission – where the child is engaged in re-enacting some aspect of the parent/care giver's traumatic experience (Ancharoff et al., 1998; Pearrow & Cosgrove, 2009).

5.6 Conclusion

Safeguarding and mental health support practices with children have developed and evolved over the past 150 years (the timespan covered in this book). New child safeguarding legislation and child protection Acts come out every couple of years, generally with the aim of strengthening safeguarding procedures, clarifying guidance and improving practices. Yet, it can be difficult to keep track of new requirements and how they impact/improve practice, also because new developments/changes are often paired with cuts to funding and resources. For example, a report by the major children's charities in the UK highlights that local authority spending on services for children and young people fell sharply between 2010 and 2018, at a time when demand for support has increased (Action for Children et al., 2018).

Alongside the sustained patterns of cuts to early intervention practices, increased spending on late intervention appears to have continued, meaning that vulnerable children and families consistently miss out on early support.

It is here, as has been argued in this chapter, that children described by Stein as 'victims' are most likely to miss out, due to their complex mental health needs and requirements. It is these children and young people who are more likely than other children to be construed as 'problematic' and 'beyond help'. Evidence of this can be found in the historic and contemporary data presented in this book, as well as from the narratives presented in the literature in this chapter. This narrative incorporates children and young people from a variety of backgrounds and cultures, young care leavers as well as child refugees – the common factor being that they are perceived as 'risky' or 'undeserving' of help for a multitude of reasons (e.g. 'difficult/bad behaviour' or 'being unchildlike', in relation to child refugees).

Here, definitions and interpretations in relation to 'childhood' as well as a 'trauma' need to be reflected upon and should take centre stage. Yet, there is also a need to rethink perceptions in relation to child safeguarding and protection; this includes reflecting on government spending priorities as it is all too easy to point the finger at 'failing disciplines and practices' whilst there is a need to look at the larger picture. In the end, it was government policy and legislation associated with the New Poor Law of 1834 (as well as the Old Poor Law of 1601) through which the notion of the 'deserving/undeserving' was introduced in the first place. This was (and still is) all too readily accepted and embraced by the middle classes – both then and now.

References

Action for Children, NCB, Children's Society, NSPCC and Barnardo's (2018). *Children and Young People's Services, Funding and Spending 2010/2011 to 2017/2018*. https://www.childrenssociety.org.uk/sites/default/files/childrens-services-funding-csfa-briefing_final.pdf.

Akister, J., Owens, M. and Goodyer, I. (2010). Leaving care and mental health: outcomes for children in out-of-home care during the transition to adulthood. *Health Research Policy and Systems*, 8, art. 10. doi:10.1186/1478-4505-8-10.

Ala, S. (2018). *The Politics of Compassion: Immigration and Asylum Policy*. Bristol: Policy Press.

Ancharoff, M.R., Munroe, J.F. and Fisher, L.M. (1998). The legacy of combat trauma: clinical implications of inter-generational transmission. In: Danieli, Y. (Ed.), *International Handbook of Multigenerational Legacies of Trauma*. New York: Plenum, 257–276.

Atherton, M. (2011). Deserving of charity or deserving of better? The continuing legacy of the 1834 Poor Law Amendment Act for Britain's deaf population. *Review of Disability Studies*, 7(3–4), 18–25.

Baldwin, J.R., Reuben, A, Newbury, J.B. and Danese, A. (2019). Agreement between prospective and retrospective measures of childhood maltreatment: a systematic review and meta-analysis. *JAMA Psychiatry*, 76(6), 584–593. doi:10.1001/jamapsychiatry.2019.0097.

Balen, R. and Masson, H. (2007). The Victoria Climbié case: social work education for practice in children and families' work before and since. *Child & Family Social Work*, 13(2), 121–132.

Baum, R. (2012). Transgenerational trauma and repetition in the body: the groove of the wound. *Body, Movement and Dance in Psychotherapy: An International Journal for Theory, Research and Practice*, 8(1), 34–42. doi:10.1080/17432979.2013.748976.

Bhaskar, R. (1989). *Reclaiming Reality*. London: Verso.

Bhaskar, R. (2014). Foreword. In: Edwards, P., O.Mahoney, J. and Vincent, S. (Eds.), *Studying Organizations Using Critical Realism: A Practical Guide*. Oxford: Oxford University Press, v–xv.

Blake, G.E.T. and Watson, E.D. (2016). Unravelling the complex mechanisms of transgenerational epigenetic inheritance. *Current Opinion in Chemical Biology*, 33, 101–107. https://www.repository.cam.ac.uk/bitstream/handle/1810/256643/Blake_et_al-2016-Current_Opinion_in_Chemical_Biology-AM.pdf?sequence=1.

Bombay, A., Matheson, K. and Anisman, H. (2014). The intergenerational effects of Indian residential schools: implications for the concept of historical trauma. *Transcultural Psychiatry*, 50(3), 320–338.

Boyden, J. (1997). Childhood and the policy makers: a comparative perspective on the globalization of childhood. In: James, A. and Prout, A. (Eds.), *Constructing and Reconstructing Childhood*. London: Routledge, 190–217.

Brown, E. (2011). The 'unchildlike child': making and marking the child/adult divide in the juvenile court. *Children's Geographies*, 9(3–4), 361–377. doi:10.1080/14733285.2011.590716.

Burchell, A. (2019). At the margins of the medical? Educational psychology, child guidance and therapy in provincial England, c.1945–1974. *Social History of Medicine*. doi:10.1093/shm/hkz097.

Carrillo, A. (2018). Using structural social work theory to drive anti-oppressive practice with Latino immigrants. *Advances in Social Work*, 18(3). doi:10.18060/21663.

Chambers, J. (2017). The neurobiology of attachment: from infancy to clinical outcomes. *Psychodynamic Psychiatry*, 45(4), 542–563. doi:10.1521/pdps.2017.45.4.542.

Choudbury, S., McKinney, K.A. and Kirmayer, J. (2015). Learning how to deal with feelings differently: psychotropic medications as vehicles of socialization in adolescence. *Social Science & Medicine*, 143, 311–319. doi:10.1016/j.socscimed.2015.02.034.

Choudbury, S. and Moses, J.M. (2016). Mindful interventions: youth, poverty, and the developing brain. *Theory & Psychology*, 26(5), 591–606.

Constantine, S. (2013) *Empire, Migration and Identity in the British World*. Manchester: Manchester University Press.

Cowan, C.S.M., Callaghan, B.L., Kan, J.M. and Richardson, R. (2016). The lasting impact of early-life adversity on individuals and their descendants: potential mechanisms and hope for intervention. *Genes, Brain and Behavior*, 15(1), 155–168.

Cowie, H. (2019). *From Birth to Sixteen: Children's Health, Social, Emotional and Linguistic Development*. London: Routledge.

Cox, P. (2013). *Bad Girls in Britain: Gender, Justice and Welfare, 1900–1950*. Basingstoke: Palgrave Macmillan.

Cradock, G. (2014). Who owns child abuse? *Social Sciences*, 3, 854–870.

Cylus, J, Roland, D, Nolte, E, Corbett, J, Jones, K, Forder, J. and Sussex, J. (2018). Identifying options for funding the NHS and social care in the UK: international evidence. Health Foundation Working Paper, 3.

de Roos, C., Greenwald, R., den Hollander-Gijsman, M., Noorthoorn, E., van Buuren, S. and de Jongh, A. (2011). A randomised comparison of cognitive behavioural therapy (CBT) and eye movement desensitisation and reprocessing (EMDR) in disaster-exposed children. *European Journal of Psychotraumatology*, 2(1). doi:10.3402/ejpt.v2i0.5694.

Delap, L. (2015). Child welfare, child protection and sexual abuse, 1918–1990. *History & Policy*. http://www.historyandpolicy.org/policy-papers/papers/child-welfare-child-protection-and-sexual-abuse-1918-1990.

Dixon, J. (2008). Young people leaving care: health, well-being and outcomes. *Child & Family Social Work*, 13, 207–217.

Duncalf, Z. (2010). *Adult Care Leavers Speak Out: The Views of 310 care leavers aged 17–78*. Manchester: Care Leavers Association.

Dziegielewski, S.F. (2016). *DSM-5 in Action*. Hoboken, NJ: Wiley (2nd edn).

Ellis, K. (2020). Blame and culpability in children's narratives of sexual abuse. *Child Abuse Review*, 28(6), 405–417.

Fisher, T, Gibbs, I, Sinclair, I and Wilson, K. (2000). Sharing the care: the qualities sought of social workers by foster carers. *Child & Family Social Work*, 5(3), 225–233.

Fong, H.-F., Alegria, M., Bair-Merritt, M.H. and Beardslee, W. (2018). Factors associated with mental health services referrals for children investigated by child welfare. *Child Abuse & Neglect*, 79, 401–412. doi:10.1016/j.chiabu.2018.01.020.

Fossion, P., Rejas, M., Servais, L., Pelc, I. and Hirsch, S. (2013). Family approach with grandchildren of Holocaust survivors. *American Journal of Psychotherapy*, 57(4), 519–527.

Frost, E., Höjer, S., Campanini, A., Sicora, A. and Kullberg, K. (2017). Why do they stay? A study of resilient child protection workers in three European countries. *European Journal of Social Work*, 21(4), 485–497. doi:10.1080/13691457.2017.1291493.

George, C. (2015). Do you have post-traumatic slave syndrome? *Ebondy*, 70(11), 67–70.

Gingell, K. (2001). The forgotten children: children admitted to a county asylum between 1854 and 1900. *Psychiatric Bulletin*, 25, 432–434.

Grenville, A. (2012). The Kindertransports: an introduction. In: Hammel, A. and Lewkowicz, B. (Eds.), *The Kindertransport to Britain 1938/39: New Perspectives*. The Yearbook of the Research Centre for German and Austrian Exile Studies, Vol. 13. Amsterdam and New York: Rodopi, 1–15.

Hacking, I. (1991). The making and molding of child abuse. *Critical Inquiry*, 17(2), 253–288.

Hall, G. Stanley (1904). *Adolescence: Its Psychology and Its Relations to Physiology, Anthropology, Sociology, Sex, Crime, Religion and Education*. New York: Appleton.

Hardwick, L. (2005). Fostering children with sexualised behaviour. *Adoption & Fostering*, 29(2), 33–43.

Hendrick, H. (1997). Constructing and reconstructing of british childhood: an interpretative survey, 1800 to the present. In: James, A. and Prout, A. (Eds.), *Constructing and Reconstructing Childhood*. London: Routledge, 34–62.

Higginbotham, P. (2017). *Children's Homes: A History of Institutional Care for Britain's Young*. Barnsley: Pen & Sword History.

Höjer, S., Frost, L., Campanini, A., Sicora, A., & Kullberg, K. (2017). Outsiders and learners: negotiating meaning in comparative European social work research practice. *Qualitative Social Work*, 16(4), 465–480. doi:10.1177/1473325015621124.

Holland, S. (2000). The assessment relationship: interactions between social workers and parents in child protection assessments. *British Journal of Social Work*, 30(2), 149–163.

Hood, R. (2014). Complexity and integrated working in children's services. *British Journal of Social Work*, 44(1), 27–43.

Hood, R. (2016). How professionals talk about complex cases: a critical discourse analysis. *Child & Family Social Work*, 21(2), 125–135. doi:10.1111? cfs.12122.

Hopkins, P. and Hill, M. (2010). The needs and strengths of unaccompanied asylum-seeking children and young people in Scotland. *Child and Family Social Work*, 15(4), 399–408.

House of Commons (2018). *Child Migration Programmes Investigation Report: Independent Inquiry Child Sexual Abuse*. https://www.gov.uk/government/p ublications, ISBN 978–971-5286–0342–3CCS0418469222 04/18.

Houston, S. (2010). Prising open the black box: critical realism, action research and social work. *Qualitative Social Work*, 9(1), 73–91. doi:10.1177/ 1473325009355622.

Hurren, E. (2015). *Protesting about Pauperism, Poverty, Politics and Poor Relief in Late-Victorian England 1870–1900*. Woodbridge: Royal Historical Society.

Jehu, L.M., Visram, S., Marks, L., Hunter, D.J., Davis, H., Mason, A., Lui, D. and Smithson, J. (2018). Directors of public health as 'a protected species':

qualitative study of the changing role of public health professionals in England following the 2013 reforms. *Journal of Public Health*, 40(3), 203–210.

Jones, T.M., Nurius, P., Song, C. and Fleming, C.M. (2018). Modeling life course pathways from adverse childhood experiences to adult mental health. *Child Abuse & Neglect*, 80, 32–40. doi:10.1016/j.chiabu.2018.03.005.

Jørgensen, M.B. and Thomson, T.L. (2018). 'Needed but undeserving': contestations of entitlement in the Danish policy framework on migration and integration. In: Fossum, J., Kastoryano, R. and Siim, B. (Eds.), *Diversity and Contestations over Nationalism in Europe and Canada*. London: Palgrave Macmillan, 337–364.

King, S.A. (2019). *Writing the Lives of the English Poor, 1750s–1830s*. Montreal: McGill-Queen's University Press.

Kinsella, M. and Monk, C. (2009). Impact of maternal stress, depression and anxiety on fetal neurobehavioural development. *Clinical Obstetrics and Gynecology*, 52(3), 425–440. doi:10.1097/GRF.0b013e3181b52df1.

Kitzinger, J. (1997). Who are you kidding? Children, power and the struggle against sexual abuse. In: James, A. and Prout, A. (Eds.), *Constructing and Reconstructing Childhood*. London: Routledge, 165–189.

Kootstra, A. (2016). Deserving and undeserving welfare claimants in Britain and the Netherlands: examining the role of ethnicity and migration status using a vignette experiment. *European Sociological Review*, 32(3), 325–338.

Kushner, T. and Knox, K. (2012). *Refugees in an Age of Genocide: Global, National and Local Perspectives during the Twentieth Century*. London: Routledge.

Leigh, K.T. and Davis, M.D. (2017). US public education: the ivy tower of historical trauma. *Journal of Philosophy & History of Education*, 67, 21–35.

Lynch, G. (2015). *Remembering Child Migration: Faith, Nation-Building and Wounds of Charity*. London: Bloomsbury.

Lynch, G. (2019). Pathways to the 1946 Curtis Report and the post-war reconstruction of children's out-of-home care. *Contemporary British History*, 34(1), 22–43.

Lyndon, S. (2019). Troubling discourses of poverty in early childhood in the UK. *Children and Society*, 33, 602–609. doi:10.1111/chso.12354.

McDonald, C. (2018). 'We became British aliens': Kindertransport refugees narrating the discovery of their parents' fates. *Holocaust Studies*, 24(4), 395–417. doi:10.1080/17504902.2018.1428784.

McLaughlin, C. (2018). 'They don't look like children': child asylum-seekers, the Dubs amendment and the politics of childhood. *Journal of Ethnic and Migration Studies*, 44(1), 1757–1773.

Melling, J., Adair, R. and Forsythe, B. (1997). 'A proper lunatic for two years': pauper lunatic children in Victorian and Edwardian England. Child Admissions to the Devon County Asylum, 1845–1914. *Journal of Social History*, 31(2), 371–394.

Memon, A., Taylor, K., Mohebati, L.M., Sundin, J., Cooper, M., Scanlon, T. and de Visser, R. (2016). Perceived barriers to accessing mental health services among black and minority ethnic (BME) communities: a qualitative study in Southeast England. *BMJ Open*, 6(11):e012337. doi:10.1136/bmjopen-2016-012337.

Morgan, M. (2020). *Care Ethics and the Refugee Crisis: Emotions, Contestation, and Agency*. New York and Abingdon: Routledge.

Morrison, J. (2016). *Familiar Strangers, Juvenile Panics and the British Press: The Decline of Social Trust*. London: Palgrave Macmillan.

Moss, E., Wildman, C., Lamont, R. and Kelly, L. (2017). Rethinking child welfare and emigration institutions, 1870–1014. *Cultural and Social History*, 14(5), 647–668.

Munro, E. (2011). *The Munro Report of Child Protection: Final Report. A Child-Centred System*. London: The Stationery Office. www.education.gov.uk/publications.

NSPCC (2016). *Children in Care: Emotional Wellbeing and Mental Health*. https://www.nspcc.org.uk/preventing-abuse/child-protection-system/children-in-care/emotional-wellbeing-of-children-in-care/.

Pearrow, M. and Cosgrove, L. (2009). The aftermath of combat-related PTSD: toward an understanding of transgenerational trauma. *Communication Disorders Quarterly*, 30(2), 77–82.

Pollock, L. (1983). *Forgotten Children: Parent–Child Relations from 1500 to 1900*. Cambridge: Cambridge University Press.

Prout, A. (2019), In defence of interdisciplinary childhood studies. *Children and Society*, 33, 309–315. doi:10.1111/chso.12298.

Prout, A. and James, A. (1997). A new paradigm for the sociology of childhood? Provenance, promise and problems. In: James, A. and Prout, A. (Eds.), *Constructing and Reconstructing Childhood*. London: Routledge, 7–33.

Rey, J.M., Assumpção, F.B., Bernad, C.A., Çuhadaroğlu, F.C., Evans, B., Fung, D., Harper, G., Loidreau, L., Ono, Y., Pūras, D., Remschmidt, H., Robertson, B., Rusakoskaya, O.A. and Schleimer, K. (2015). History of child and adolescent psychiatry. In: Rey, J.M. (Ed.), *IACAPAP e-Textbook of Child and Adolescent Mental Health*. Geneva: International Association for Child and Adolescent Psychiatry and Allied Professions, 1–67.

Sales, R. (2002). The deserving and the undeserving? Refugees, asylum seekers and welfare in Britain. *Critical Social Policy*, 22(3), 456–478.

Sharf, R. (2014). Mindfulness and mindlessness in early Chan. *Philosophy East and West* 64(4), 933–964.

Sims-Schouten, W. and Edwards, S. (2016). 'Man up!' Bullying and resilience within a neoliberal framework. *Journal of Youth Studies*, 19(10), 1382–1400.

Sims-Schouten, W. and Hayden, C., (2017). Mental health and wellbeing of care leavers: making sense of their perspectives. *Child & Family Social Work*, 24(4), 1480–1487.

Sims-Schouten, W. and Riley, S.E. (2014). Employing a form of critical realist discourse analysis for identity research: an example from women's talk of motherhood, childcare and employment. In: Edwards, P., O'Mahoney, J. and

Vincent, S. (Eds.), *Studying Organizations Using Critical Realism: A Practical Guide*. Oxford: Oxford University Press, 46–65.

Sims-Schouten, W., Skinner, A. and Rivett, K. (2019). Child safeguarding in light of the deserving/undeserving paradigm: a historical and contemporary analysis. *Child Abuse & Neglect*, 94. doi:10.1016/j.chiabu.2019.104025.

Slack, K. and Webber, M. (2008). Do we care? Adult mental health professionals' attitudes towards supporting service users' children. *Child & Family Social Work*, 13(1), 72–79.

Spyrou, S. (2019). An ontological turn for childhood studies? *Children & Society*, 33, 316–323. doi:10.1111/chso.12292.

Steffel, M., William, E.F. and Perrmann-Graham, J. (2016). Passing the buck: delegating choices to others to avoid responsibility and blame. *Organizational Behavior and Human Decision Processes*, 135, 32–44.

Stein, E. (2000). *Philosophy of Psychology and the Humanities*. Washington: ICS Publications.

Stein, M. (2006). Research review: young people leaving care, *Child and Family Social Work*, 11(3), 273–279.

Stryker, R., Boddy, J., Bragg, S. and Sims-Schouten, W. (2019). The future of childhood studies and Children & Society. *Children & Society*, 33, 301–308. doi:10.1111/chso.12345.

Thane, P. (2012). The 'big society' and the 'big state': creative tension or crowding out? *Twentieth Century British History*, 23, 408–429.

Thomas, N. (2019). What is the point of studying childhood as a social phenomenon? *Children & Society*, 33, 324–332. doi:10.1111/chso.12297.

Tisdall, E.K.M. (2017) Conceptualising children and young people's participation: examining vulnerability, social accountability and co-production. *International Journal of Human Rights*, 21(1), 59–75. doi:10.1080/13642987. 2016.1248125.

Turpel-Lafond, M.E. (2014). *Lost in the Shadows: How a Lack of Help Meant a Loss of Hope for One First Nations Girl. Investigative Report*. Victoria, BC: Representative for Children and Youth. https://rcybc.ca/sites/default/ files/documents/pdf/reports_publications/rcy_lost-in-the-shadows_forweb_ 17feb.pdf.

Ungar, M. (2002). *Playing at Being Bad: The Hidden Resilience of Troubled Teens*. Halifax, NS: Pottersfield Press.

Ungar, M. (2004). *Nurturing Hidden Resilience in Troubled Youth*. Toronto: University of Toronto Press.

Ungar, M. (2005). *A Handbook for Working with Children and Youth: Pathways to Resilience across Cultures and Contexts*. Thousand Oaks, CA: Sage.

Van Keer, R.L., Deschepper, R, Huyghens. and Bilsen, J. (2017). Mental well-being of patients from ethnic minority groups during critical care: a qualitative ethnographic study. *BMJ Open*, 7. doi:10.1136/bmjopen-2016-014075.

Waechter, R., Kumanayaka, D. and Angus-Yamada, C. (2019). Maltreatment history, trauma symptoms and research reactivity among adolescents in child protection services. *Child and Adolescent Psychiatry and MentalHealth*, 13(13). doi:10.1186/s13034-019-0270-7.

Whittaker, A. and Havard, A. (2015). Defensive practice as 'fear-based' practice: social work's open secret? *British Journal of Social Work*, 46(5), 1158–1174. doi:10.1093/bjsw/bcv048.

Woodcock Ross, J. (2016). *Specialist Communication Skills for Social Workers: Developing Professional Capability*. London: Palgrave (2nd edn).

Wynter, R. (2015). Pictures of Peter Pan: institutions, local definitions of 'mental deficiency', and the filtering of children in early twentieth-century England. *Family & Community History*, 18(2), 122–138. doi:10.1179/1463118015Z.00000000045.

Zarse, E.M., Neff, M.R., Yoder, R., Hulvershorn, L., Chambers, J.E. and Chambers, A.R. (2019). The adverse childhood experiences questionnaire: two decades of research on childhood trauma as a primary cause of adult mental illness, addiction, and medical diseases. *Cogent Medicine*, 6(1), doi:10.1080/2331205X.2019.1581447.

Conclusion

Changing perceptions: a way forward

There is no doubt that measures to promote child welfare have developed and evolved over the past 150 years. However, to an extent, the way in which safeguarding, wellbeing and mental health in childhood are approached today mirrors practices and perceptions of the late 19th century, particularly in relation to 'vulnerable groups' of people, such as children in care and young care leavers. By 'vulnerable' I mean individuals or groups of individuals who are made vulnerable by the situations and environments they are exposed to, rather than through any inherent weakness or lack of capacity. This book has shown how looked after children, care leavers and their families were and are frequently positioned within a lower social class/hierarchy, and stigmatised as less important than other children/families. Moreover, the research in this book highlights how the 'beyond help' narrative seems to be reserved for the children and young people with the most complex needs, and related behavioural and mental health issues. It is these particularly vulnerable children who end up being judged and held accountable for their 'bad' behaviour.

The purpose of this book and the related research was to engage in a critical reflection of the ideals and rationales of historic and contemporary child safeguarding and mental health support practices, and the legacy of the deserving/undeserving paradigm here. This also means engaging with challenges in relation to conflicting research findings and experiences, which need to be placed in context. For example, while on the one hand the state of affairs in residential homes for children, both historically and in contemporary times, has been described in terms of utter loneliness and lacking in care and support, there are also accounts of the more supportive nature of children's homes and institutions (Care of Children Committee, 1946; Moss et al., 2017). Moreover, while some stress the altruistic motives behind the child rescue movement of the late 1800s and current support schemes for displaced and disadvantaged children and young people, others show a more sinister story of abuse, bad treatment and racism (Cradock, 2014; Hacking, 1991; Lynch, 2019; Roberts-Pichette, 2016).

The data presented in this book shows that, in light of stigmas as well as budget cuts and caps on resources, decisions tend to be made about who can or can't be helped. For example, the notion of a child being 'beyond help' appeared in 46 per cent of the historic children's case files discussed in Chapter 3 and in 50 per cent of the interviews with practitioners in the contemporary dataset presented in Chapter 4. Yet, it should be noted that it is not only vulnerable children and families who are disadvantaged by uneven and unequal provision of services – changing thresholds and cuts to services also affect staff who are committed to helping and supporting those in their care. It is here that critical realist ontology is useful in making sense of differentiated and stratified social structures, as well as the quandary between three structural concepts: 'absence' (under-representation, under-privilege and what is missing in a context or institution/organisation highlighting a possible need for a critical focus); 'difference' (stigma and labels in relation to 'bad behaviour' and mental illness); and 'threat' (e.g. high cost of services, 'immoral behaviour') (Chauhan & Foster, 2014; Roberts & Schiavenato, 2017). All of the above is exacerbated by the COVID-19 pandemic.

In the Introduction to this book I stated that I felt indebted to the young people and practitioners who were part of my research, and that all of them have left their mark and my heart goes out to them. It is here, with them, that we need to start when it comes to changing perceptions, working our way through the maze of sometimes confusing, stigmatising and contradictory practices and perceptions. There is a need to centralise young people's needs/voices in decisions around services that affect them. Better identification of young people at risk of developing PTSD is needed, and intervening early to treat mental health conditions can help minimise the wide range of negative impacts on young people's lives. Evidence suggests that two sets of factors are of key importance in understanding the risk and protective factors shaping the mental health of young people following trauma exposure, as well as being potential portals for interventions: exposure to past and ongoing traumatic events; and the complexities of navigating support systems/environments, including dealing with school and reconfigured family life (Waechter et al., 2019; Zarse et al., 2019).

My previous research (Sims-Schouten & Hayden, 2017) highlights the value of engaging with (young) people in understanding their needs and developing systems of formal/informal support. Yet, despite calls for greater involvement of young people in services that affect them, in reality this is often tokenistic or a 'tick box' exercise. What is needed is a framework that centralises the needs and voices of the most vulnerable young people in our societies, and developing practice and conceptualisations around factors that cause and maintain trauma. These include: abuse, neglect and transitions (the 'real' level); individual experiences and capabilities therein (the 'empirical' level); and the formal/informal support systems currently in place, as well as gaps in this area (the 'actual'). Applied critical realism (CR) provides possible answers to this, which will be discussed further in the next section.

Applying CR and making sense of mental health and safeguarding in childhood

Drawing on critical realism, my starting point is that perceptions of mental health and safeguarding in childhood are tied to and a product of individual experiences and social contexts (and related interpretations) of inequality/complexity, e.g. in relation to trauma/stress, affecting children and young people differently across time and space. Current mental health interventions are limited by adopting partial understandings and reductionist ideas of health, pathology, 'normality' and personhood. In part, these challenges occur because mental health/mental illness are contested terms, used to represent a range of concepts from psychological states to dimensions of health (Patel & Pilgrim, 2018; Pilgrim, 2015). For example, psychiatric models hold the premise that mental illness has an external reality that can be subsequently identified by experts, whilst approaches drawing on social and constructionist models tend to infer that we can only know the world via the ways we represent it (Cromby & Harper, 2009; Pilgrim, 2014). Both models are limited in their ability to cater for the needs of vulnerable children with complex needs, either by being too reductionist (biomedical models) or too relativist (social models).

Critical realism, and its focus on inferential reasoning, allows for a critique of the way in which mental health issues are conceptualised, and instead turns to the conditions under which variations in behaviour and the expression of distress are described in one way rather than another (Bhaskar, 1989, 2014; Sims-Schouten & Riley, 2014). Taking a critical realist lens allowed the analysis to be contextualised within (non-linear) causal patterns and effects, for example, the power of institutions in different eras (and related thresholds and perceptions), as well as the material contexts and social position of the participants (see also Sims-Schouten et al., 2019). Thus, drawing on critical realist ontology, I was able to explore some of the complexities in relation to: causal factors (referred to as the 'real'); how things in relation to neglect, abuse, mental health issues and related support are experienced (the 'empirical'); and what process and support systems are in place (the 'actual'). Taking this further, the research presented in this book has identified potential causal events (material, institutional or embodied) that may produce experienced events (such as being marginalised). This in turn can be accounted for from both an experiential standpoint (i.e. how it made the participant vulnerable) and an accountability standpoint (leading to judgements from practitioners about 'worthiness' and 'deservedness'), which also needs to be seen in light of cuts to services and changing thresholds for support.

This has implications for practice, and the research presented in this book sheds light on historic and contemporary uneven safeguarding practices and related subjective distinctions between those who are 'deserving' and 'undeserving' (e.g. in relation to perceived behaviour and lifestyle choices), calling for more reflectivity and reflexivity in working with vulnerable children and families. In practice this means engaging with children and young people's stories, experiences and realities on three levels: first, the 'real' level, namely causal factors such as trauma and stress; second, the 'empirical' level, namely how mental health problems are experienced by the children and young people, also in relation to stigma; third, the 'actual' level, namely events and processes that occur and are in place in relation to safeguarding mental health support. Here, not only do we need to zoom in on the experiences and children and young people; we also need to understand how support systems are organised (or not) as it is not only vulnerable children and families who suffer here. Despite examples of failure in practice, most staff involved in the protection of children are committed to helping and supporting those in their care. This is negatively affected by ongoing cuts to services, staff shortages and a lack of time to spend with families (Sims-Schouten, 2020).

References

Bhaskar, R. (1989). *Reclaiming Reality*. London: Verso.

Bhaskar, R. (2014). Foreword. In: Edwards, P., O.Mahoney, J. and Vincent. S. (Eds.), *Studying Organizations Using Critical Realism: A Practical Guide*. Oxford: Oxford University Press, v–xv.

Care of Children Committee (1946). *Report of the Care of Children Committee.* London: HMSO.

Chauhan, A. and Foster, J. (2014). Representations of poverty in British newspapers: a case of 'othering' the threat? *Journal of Community and Applied Social Psychology,* 24(5), 390–405.

Cradock, G. (2014). Who owns child abuse? *Social Sciences,* 3, 854–870.

Cromby, J. and Harper, D.J. (2009). Paranoia: a social account. *Theory & Psychology,* 19(3), 335–361. doi:10.1177/0959354309104158.

Hacking, I. (1991), The making and molding of child abuse. *Critical Inquiry,* 17(2), 253–288.

Lynch, G. (2019). Pathways to the 1946 Curtis Report and the post-war reconstruction of children's out-of-home care. *Contemporary British History,* 34(1), 22–43.

Moss, E., Wildman, C., Lamont, R. and Kelly, L. (2017). Rethinking child welfare and emigration institutions, 1870–1014. *Cultural and Social History,* 14(5), 647–668.

Patel, N. and Pilgrim, D. (2018). Psychologists and torture: critical realism as a resource for analysis and training. *Journal of Critical Realism,* 7(2), 176–191.

Pilgrim, D. (2014). Some implications of critical realism for mental health research. *Social Theory & Health,* 12(1), 1–12.

Pilgrim, D. (2015). The Biopsychosocial model in health research: its strengths and limitations for critical realists. *Journal of Critical Realism,* 14(2), 164–180.

Roberts, M.L.M. and Schiavenato, M. (2017). Othering in the nursing context: a concept analysis. *Nursing Open,* 4, 174–181.

Roberts-Pichette, P. (2016). *Great Canadian Expectations: The Middlemore Experience.* Carleton Place, Ontario: Global Heritage Press.

Sims-Schouten, W. and Hayden, C., (2017). Mental health and wellbeing of care leavers: making sense of their perspectives. *Child & Family Social Work,* 24(4), 1480–1487.

Sims-Schouten, W. and Riley, S.E. (2014). Employing a form of critical realist discourse analysis for identity research: An example from women's talk of motherhood, childcare and employment. In: Edwards, P., O'Mahoney, J. and Vincent, S. (Eds.), *Studying Organizations Using Critical Realism: A Practical Guide.* Oxford: Oxford University Press, 46–65.

Sims-Schouten, W. (2020). Victorian attitudes can still be found in child protection services today. *The Conversation.* https://theconversation.com/victorian-attitudes-can-still-be-found-in-child-protection-services-today-129510.

Sims-Schouten, W., Skinner, A. and Rivett, K. (2019). Child safeguarding in light of the deserving/undeserving paradigm: a historical and contemporary analysis. *Child Abuse & Neglect,* 94. doi:10.1016/j.chiabu.2019.104025.

Waechter, R., Kumanayaka, D. and Angus-Yamada, C. (2019). Maltreatment history, trauma symptoms and research reactivity among adolescents in child protection services, *Child and Adolescent Psychiatry and MentalHealth,* 13(13). doi:10.1186/s13034-019-0270-7.

Zarse, E.M., Neff, M.R., Yoder, R., Hulvershorn, L., Chambers, J.E. and Chambers, A.R. (2019). The adverse childhood experiences questionnaire: two decades of research on childhood trauma as a primary cause of adult mental illness, addiction, and medical diseases. *Cogent Medicine*, 6(1). doi:10.1080/2331205X.2019.1581447.

Index

Page numbers in bold refer to tables.